Yoga for Kids to Teens

Praise for Yoga for Kids to Teens

"Lots of studies show how much we all need to exercise and to reduce our stress. And this is even true for our youngest citizens. Luckily the authors have created a great guide for learning not only yoga poses but also for understanding the deeper truths upon which yoga is based. Highly recommended for teachers of this special age group."

—Judith Hanson Lasater, PhD, PT.
Author of 30 *Essential Yoga Poses* and *A Year of Living Your Yoga*.

"Yael, Matthew, and Nicole have crafted a warm, insightful, and playful companion to their previous offering, *Create a Yoga Practice for Kids*. Yael shares her solid background in asana with liberal sprinkles of wisdom and whimsy. Matthew offers kids a lovely glimpse into their inner worlds, giving them skills they can use throughout their lives. Nicole's innovative Stikk Yoga is creative, interactive, and just plain fun!"

—Charlotte Bell, E-RYT. Author of *Mindful Yoga, Mindful Life* (Rodmell, 2007).

"This book should be on the shelf wherever children and young adults gather. Clear, creative instruction offers many opportunities to learn and teach yoga. From meditation and relaxation, slow flow to intense asana, there is much information here."

—Marsha Wenig, Founder, YogaKids® International.

"Whether you are a parent, teacher or youth, you'll love this book because it's so easy to use, filled with fun facts, creative yoga sequences, child-centered techniques, ready-to-use scripts for thematic lessons, with meaningful quotes and questions to ponder. I am inspired by the richness of this text and the authenticity of yoga for kids it expresses such as the importance of breath, body awareness, proper alignment, relaxation, self-discovery and positivity."

—Jodi B. Komitor, MA, RYT, Author of *The Complete Idiot's Guide to Yoga with Kids* and Founder of Next Generation Yoga.

"Yael, Matthew, and Nicole have given yoga teachers everywhere a great gift and a loving reminder in Yoga for Kids to Teens. Through their creativity and lightness of being, they bring the joy back into the practice, reminding us not to take ourselves or yoga too seriously..."

—Linda Sparrowe, author of *A Woman's Book of Yoga and Health: A Lifelong Guide to Wellness* (Shambhala, 2002) and Editor-in-Chief of *Natural Solutions* magazine.

"It is thanks to books like this that the true gifts of Yoga are so readily available to all children. *Yoga For Kids to Teens* shows us ease, teaches us innovation, and leads us into the very heart of Yoga itself. Without watering down the discipline, the authors give the youth of today permission to become innovators and participants in their own lives..."

—D'ana Baptiste, owner of Centered City Yoga in Salt Lake City.

"There are so many great innovative ideas expressed in this book, from imaginative ways to instruct young students, to the SOLA Stikk for extending the yoga experience. As a scientist, I resonated with the instruction to encourage students to become scientists and observe how their bodies respond with each new action. The inspired efforts of these authors will surely guide the emergence of many new yogi scientists!"
—David H. Bradshaw, PhD, Dept. of Anesthesiology, University of Utah.

"This book is a gem, full of creative and thoughtful ways to introduce youth to yoga in a broad reaching manner that is sure to bring valuable life skills into their lives…In addition to tips for teaching, it weaves benefits of poses, artistic expression, physical anatomy, playfulness, the value of setting intentions, as well as exploring the breath and medication into detailed lesson plans."
—Trace Michelle Childress, Program Coordinator, Omega Institute, New York.

"This is a book I will turn to again and again. The instruction is engaging, clear, creative and individually empowering. It gives anyone, yoga novice or experienced yoga teacher, the tools to make teaching yoga to children easy and fun. And it offers children permission to celebrate their bodies, whatever size or shape they may be."
—Elizabeth Finlinson, LCSW, Salt Lake City.

"*Yoga for Kids to Teens* is fascinating and informative, but above all delightful. It is a treasure trove of information about yoga for students of all types. It is especially useful for those who teach children and people with special needs. A wonderful book that belongs on the bookshelf—no, in the hands—of every yoga practitioner and teacher."
—Michael Goldfield, Founder, Yoga for Stiff People.

"I am thrilled to finally find a current children's yoga book that makes practicing yoga safe, fun, and simple. This is an amazing tool for educators and even parents, looking to introduce yoga into their children's lives. I have been using this as a tool to instruct educators and teachers just love it! I can't say enough wonderful things about this book!"
—Cindy Valentine, MEd.

"*Yoga for Kids to Teens* is an excellent resource for anyone who wants to share yoga with children. It is user-friendly, straight-forward, full of relevant themes, facts and tips as well as great coaching from an experienced teacher."
—Leah Kalish, Program Director, YogaED.

"I know our yoga teachers could certainly use this book as a tool!"
—Jennifer Wert, Deputy Director, The Wellness Initiative, Denver, Colorado.

Yoga for Kids to Teens

Themes, Relaxation Techniques, Games
and an Introduction to SOLA Stikk Yoga

by
Yael Calhoun
and
Matthew R. Calhoun
and
Nicole M. Hamory

Illustrated by Carol Anne Coogan

SUNSTONE
PRESS

SANTA FE

Sunstone books may be purchased for educational, business, or sales promotional use. For information please write: Special Markets Department, Sunstone Press, P.O. Box 2321, Santa Fe, New Mexico 87504-2321.

Book design » Vicki Ahl
Body typeface » Verdana
Printed on acid free paper

Library of Congress Cataloging-in-Publication Data

Calhoun, Yael.
  Yoga for kids to teens : themes, relaxation techniques, games and an introduction to Sola Stikk(tm) yoga / by Yael Calhoun, Matthew R. Calhoun and Nicole Hamory ; illustrated by Carol Anne Coogan.
    p. cm.
  ISBN 978-0-86534-686-4 (softcover : alk. paper)
  1. Hatha yoga for children--Handbooks, manuals, etc. 2. Hatha yoga for teenagers--Handbooks, manuals, etc. I. Calhoun, Matthew R. II. Hamory, Nicole. III. Title.
  RA781.7.C354 2008
  613.7'046--dc22
                                            2008038010

Published in

WWW.SUNSTONEPRESS.COM
SUNSTONE PRESS / POST OFFICE BOX 2321 / SANTA FE, NM 87504-2321 /USA
(505) 988-4418 / ORDERS ONLY (800) 243-5644 / FAX (505) 988-1025

To all of my family:
the roots, the trunk, the branches, and the leaves.
—Yael Calhoun

One has many teachers in life; too few great ones.
My main teacher of Yoga has been Lilias Folan, who spoke to
me through her television shows, books, videos, CD's, and in
recent years in person through her classes. Her special talent and
generosity have made Yoga a more loving experience for me,
and for that, may she be twice blessed.
—Matthew Calhoun

SOLA Yoga Stikk is dedicated to all the potential yoga students
who have always wanted to try yoga but didn't think they could.
My section of the book is especially for you.
—Nicole Hamory

If I am not for myself, who will be for me?
If I am not for others, what am I?
And if not now, when?
—Hillel

CONTENTS

ACKNOWLEDGEMENTS

A book is a reflection of one's thoughts and passions, which are shaped by experiences. I feel much gratitude toward my first yoga teacher, Charlotte Bell, who for years created a yoga environment in which I could learn and explore. For sharing and exploring the yoga vision, I am grateful to my coauthors, Matthew, the inscrutable wizard, and Nicole, the boundless well of creativity and goodness. I would like to thank Judith Hanson Lasater, Lilias Folan, and Donna Farhi, whose books and workshops have helped to shape my yoga practice and teaching. I have had the good fortune to study with some dedicated yoga teachers, including the inspiring Adam Ballenger and uplifting Joanne Payne. And, as importantly, I thank all of those students, in many settings and of many ages, that have provided me the opportunity to teach and to therefore learn for over 25 years. This book would not be nearly as fun without the bountiful patience and talent of our wonderful illustrator, Carol Anne Coogan. And a warm thank you to Dr. Timothy McCall and Richard Rosen, who honored our efforts to share yoga by reading our work.

Special thanks to Elizabeth Finlinson, friend extraordinaire, for the many hours of yoga practice and discussions in a sunny room overlooking all seasons in the Rocky Mountains. Aram Calhoun—one sustained (and sustainable) thank you for too many reasons to list. And of course, I want to thank my sons—Alex, Ben, and Sam, who taught many yoga classes with me this summer and made sure the themes were kid friendly. Their standard is simple—if it is not fun, don't do it. And a very heartfelt thanks to my husband, Patrick A. Tresco, who made sure this book had whatever it needed to grow. Finally, thanks to Ima Panim and my father, for the deep roots from which this grew.

—Yael Calhoun

There is so much gratitude to express for the vision, creation and follow through that evolved through this book. Firstly, my co-author and co-creator of GreenTREE Yoga, Yael Calhoun. Integrity, vision, focus and patience—words can't express how much I appreciate you and your family!

Secondly, my family: Dad, Mom, Alex, Majanne and Marlis—for all the creativity we shared as a family. Thirdly, Mark Phillips, for teaching me the importance of integrity, confidence, and kindness. Lastly, to all my students everywhere—always an honor and a pleasure to watch you shine! Thank you for your willingness to learn and fall in love with Yoga!

—Nicole Hamory

I. INTRODUCTION

*One's mind, once stretched by a new idea,
never regains its original dimensions.*
—Oliver Wendell Holmes

The Book

This book expands the kids' yoga developed in our first book, *Create a Yoga Practice for Kids: Fun Flexibility and Focus* (Sunstone Press, 2006), while it also introduces the new "Five Minute Yoga Classroom Break" and the energizing SOLA Stikk Yoga. Many people now want yoga ideas for 'tweens and teens, so this book addresses a wider audience, as we include youth to young adults and have added "Challenge" sections. Our purpose is to share ways to give people yoga as a life long learning tool and to expose them to a wonderful way to make themselves both emotionally and physically stronger.

This book has three sections, each reflecting the individual author's unique style of teaching and asana practice. Each of us invites you to create your own yoga practice by weaving together different sections to meet the needs of your group—whether it be kids, teens, high school athletes, or people with special needs.

1. The first section contains new themes and yoga games developed by Yael in her teaching of kids' yoga to diverse populations in a variety of settings: schools, libraries, shelters, and summer camps. The themes are interactive and sure to keep everyone's attention as they move and laugh their way toward a good yoga practice. Yael develops themes based on a topic in which everyone has an interest—their own bodies. Sharing yoga in this way keeps the yoga dynamic and interesting for all ages.

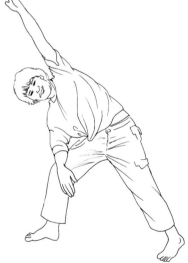

This section also introduces the "The Five Minute Classroom Yoga Break", a section requested by teachers both as a classroom management tool and to help them meet some state PE requirements. It is designed for use in grades K-12. A CD is also available: Yoga for Kids and Classroom (Greentree Yoga, 2008)

2. The second section of the book offers more of Matthew's "mind/body" yoga games, meditations and relaxation exercises. Integrated into a yoga journey, poses are used to invite meditation and healing into a practice. Youth comes with a supple body and open mind. A major benefit of yoga is to teach us to release the mental and physical stress and tension of modern living. To teach a young person to learn with a relaxed mind and body is to offer a gift that can last a lifetime.

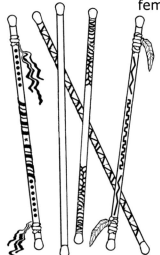

3. The third section brings us back to energizing yoga, as we proudly and happily introduce the all new and engaging SOLA Stikk, developed by Nicole to add support and artistic expression to a practice. Nicole thought of using a stick as a yoga prop as she was cross-country skiing in the Rocky Mountains one winter's day and began to use her ski pole to do some yoga stretches. The SOLA Stikk was developed to help people hold poses longer, find intuitive alignment, and deepen their stretches. The SOLA Stikk can also serve as an individual totem, or an artistic expression of qualities or values one wants to incorporate into everyday life. SOLA Stikk yoga is a wonderful approach to engage every age and ability level—from kids to high school athletes to people with physical or emotional challenges. SOLA is an acronym for (S) Self-awareness, (O) Observation, (L) Love and (A) Acceptance. SOLA Yoga is program developed by Nicole during her years of teaching yoga to college students, youth at risk, cancer survivors, and male and female prisoners.

SOLA Stikks

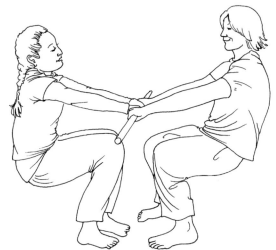

SOLA Stikk Trusting Squat

What is Yoga?

*There's only one corner of the universe
you can be certain of improving,
and that's yourself.
—Aldous Huxley*

Perhaps the first question should be why, in a nation obsessed by youth, are almost 16 million Americans doing yoga, an art and science that is thousands of years old? The answer is simple. Yoga is growing in popularity as people experience it as a wonderfully effective tool for making positive changes in our bodies, our minds, and our lives. Yoga has many proven benefits, which are now being studied by Western scientists.

And yoga is not a one-size-fit-all-idea. Part of the growing appeal of yoga is that it is not one dimensional. Yoga is not just a sitting meditation or just a practice of energizing, challenging poses. There are so many styles of yoga (Hatha, Iyengar, Ashtanga, Anusara, Viniyoga, Kundaline, and Bikram to name but a few), and from this we can find an approach that fits our specific needs for the day, the week, or the year. As Lilias Folan notes in her inspiring book, *Lilias! Yoga Gets Better With Age,* "Yoga is a vehicle for inner growth and development. It can be adapted to fit every body, no matter what size, shape, age, or physical condition—all are welcome!"[1]

So what is yoga? There are various interpretations of the word. One is yoking or union, a coming together. It can be as simple as forming a union as your hands touch the mat, or a more interesting union as when you "feel" or experience a connection between the mind and the body. Another interpretation discussed by Desikachar is that yoga is a process toward achieving what was previously unattainable.[2] So any action we take, any movement we make, toward what we want to achieve, is yoga.

For many, the heart of yoga is based on Patanjali's *Yoga Sutras,* a work that put in writing the ancient teachings of yoga. The Yoga Sutras, written about 2,000 years ago, deal with all aspects of the human condition. Yoga is not a religion, but a way of moving through life, compatible with any spiritual belief system. As Charlotte Bell explains in her informative and accessible book, *Mindful Yoga, Mindful Life,* the meaning of yoga is captured in Patanjali's second aphorism, itself subject to various interpretations. A translation meaningful to her is that of Alistair Shearer: Yoga Sutra 1.2: "Yoga is the settling of the mind into silence."[3]

And so, again, yoga is definitely not a religion. It is a way using our senses—our minds and our bodies—to explore ourselves and our world in a more positive and productive way. As B.K.S. Iyengar, one of the world's leading teachers of yoga, offers: "Yoga is a fine art and seeks to express the artist's abilities to the fullest possible extent. While most artists need an instrument to express their art, the only instruments a yogi needs are his body and his mind."[4]

What Does Yoga Offer Kids and Teens?

> In the beginner's mind there are many
> possibilities, in the expert's mind there are few.
> —Suzuki Roshi

1. Yoga is fun:

Yoga works with kids and teens for some very simple reasons. One is that yoga can be fun and can allow people the opportunity to smile and laugh. The fun factor, which provides an opportunity to connect with people, is a key because it lowers stress levels in the body so people want to keep doing it. Doing yoga makes people smile. Smiling is contagious owing to people's tendency to mimic the mood or expression of those around them, as explained in the book *Emotional Contagion*. Smiling not only improves people's frame of mind, but it also can improve the quality of personal interactions.[5]

2. Yoga promotes self-discovery:

Judith Hanson Lasater notes that yoga is a journey to self-discovery[6]. And who are, or should be, more actively involved in self discovery than young people? As kids and teens continually strive to develop and to define who they are, yoga gives them a powerful tool with which to explore both themselves and their world. They can develop a more positive outlook, more confidence, and more physical and mental strength. In addition, yoga provides kids and teens with an opportunity to explore who they are in a noncompetitive, supportive environment.

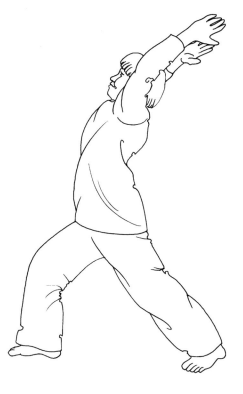

3. Yoga fosters social interaction and team building:

Yoga, and the laughter and smiles it generates, can be used as a team building activity or to encourage understanding between diverse groups. Social interaction and group dynamics are highly important to kids and teens. Science has shown us that shared laughter increases a sense of closeness among people, which is a step toward understanding.[7] Daniel Goleman, in his book *Social Intelligence*, discusses the biological effect of smiling, improving people's moods and outlooks. He states that "laughter may be the shortest distance between two brains, an unstoppable infectious spread that builds an instant social bond."[8]

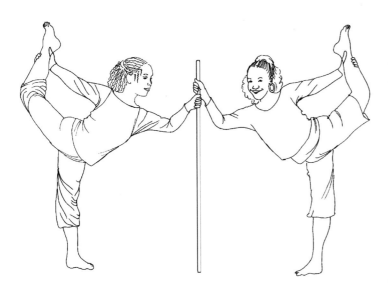

4. Yoga addresses risk factors:

Consider this insight from a male prisoner who regularly attends one of Nicole's prison yoga classes. The day after the Virginia Tech shootings (4/16/07), he said, "That guy really needed to do yoga."

Yoga programs address risk factors such as substance abuse, violence, and social isolation that challenge many populations for many reasons. Yoga engages people in physical exercise and develops concentration and focus. Yoga also builds trust, self-confidence and positive feelings, fosters creativity and exercises the imagination, and improves the learning environment.

5. Yoga decreases stress:

The human race has only one really effective weapon, and that is laughter.
—Mark Twain

A major benefit of yoga is that it decreases stress and

teaches people how to do simple relaxation techniques. We know that our youth is under increasing amounts of social stress, emotional stress, and physical stress. Yoga decreases stress through the physical release of the muscles, the building of positive self image, and also through learning to work with the breath. Yoga breathing and breath awareness helps to decrease heart rate, decrease blood pressure, and decrease stress hormone levels in the body.

In his book, *Yoga as Medicine: The Yogic Prescription for Health and Healing* (Bantam, 2007), Dr. Timothy McCall outlines the many ways in which yoga decreases stress levels, giving us scientific data to support such claims. In addition, he identifies the many health risks associated with heightened stress levels, including diabetes, obesity, heart disease, and depression to name but a few. At Needham High School in Massachusetts, the principal has scheduled yoga classes for all seniors as part of their stress reduction program.[9] One seven year-old said to Yael after a class, "I have a lot of yoga DVDs at home, but none makes me feel this relaxed." It had, interestingly, been a very active class, yet she felt calmer at the end of it.

6. Yoga is flexible:

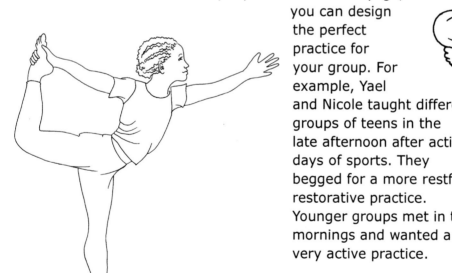

Because there are many styles and facets to yoga, you can design the perfect practice for your group. For example, Yael and Nicole taught different groups of teens in the late afternoon after active days of sports. They begged for a more restful, restorative practice. Younger groups met in the mornings and wanted a very active practice.

Easy Pose

Standing Bow

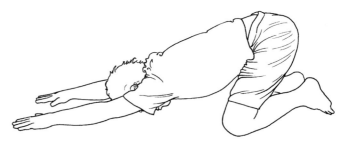

Extended Child's Pose

Nicole works with one group of high school athletes who loves yoga. As a high school senior at West High in Salt Lake City says, "Yoga is absolutely, phenomically amazing! It helps me discipline my body and to find my inner strength. It prepares me for school and the future. I wish I could do it everyday. Hail to yoga!"[10]

So anywhere you have kids and teens, there are many opportunities to use yoga, to let yoga works its magic.

Imagine That!

Visualize this thing that you want, see it, feel it, believe in it. Make your mental blue print, and begin to build.
—*Robert Collier*

Practicing yoga provides an opportunity to practice a powerful healing tool—visualization. Science has shown us that visualizing, or imagining, doing something or thinking in a positive way can produce a physiological change in the brain. That is to say, the action of a thought can actually change the path the neurons follow when they fire. Think about how a golfer or a baseball player takes a few practice swings before executing the shot. They are using both the mind and the body to perfect an action.

The idea of visualizing to make something happen can be taught. Yael had a seven year old boy from the Sudan in a class. She was speaking about looking up and seeing the clouds. He interrupted her, saying, "But there are no clouds". She agreed, but explained that you could imagine the clouds up there as you lifted your head and stretched toward the sky. She watched him as he closed his eyes. Now as he did the exercise, a huge smile spread over his face. He had, Yael thought, just gained a new tool.

Nischala Joy Devi explains in *The Healing Path of Yoga* that imagery can be used to actively create a situation or form an idea in one's mind. One can imagine different senses (seeing, hearing, tasting, feeling) to develop images in the mind. Guiding children through simple visualization exercises introduces them to ways they can find their own state of relaxation.

Here is one easy, yet powerful, way to introduce the idea of visualization to people. At the beginning of the practice, as you all sit with eyes closed, invite everyone to imagine a peaceful scene with them in it (even give some ideas). Then pause and give them time to find that place in their minds. Then, at the end of the practice, as everyone is sitting or lying quietly, ask them to visualize themselves doing what they would like to do in life—in college, finding a career they enjoy, pursing a dream they have. Again, pause and give them a few moments to ponder this point of success and achievement. Such a simple activity can plant some seeds for success, which hopefully future yoga practices or other activities will nurture.

Many of these exercises in this book contain ideas for helping to practice visualization. We invite you to offer this gift to both yourself and the people with whom you are sharing yoga. Imagine that!

Where do I begin?

> *All serious daring starts from within.*
> *—Eudora Welty*

A good starting point for practicing yoga is the decision that you want to do something positive for yourself—both mind and body. So begin on a yoga mat with an open mind, coming with the attitude that you are there to see what yoga has to offer. Leave any expectations or judgments in another place. Bring only your ability to observe what is happening with you—your body and your mind. After just one practice or class, most people feel better. Even if they cannot say exactly why, they know the effect is positive. And that is the beginning.

We work with some people for just one class, while others have the opportunity for a more consistent practice over the year. But even one class, one opportunity to experience, to *feel* yoga can be enough to inspire people to find another class, to get a DVD or a book, or to practice with a mom or a friend. Kids will often say after one class, I am going to do yoga with my grandma now, or my aunt has a DVD and I am going to do it with her. Parents who come to a family yoga class for their kids will often say that they are now going to seek out an adult class.

And from that starting point, with time and practice, one can do more, learn more, experience more, and just allow oneself to *be* more.

Challenging Poses and Variations

One can never consent to creep when one feels an impulse to soar.
—Helen Keller

By popular request, we have added a "Challenge" section to many poses, as well as variations. For the challenging poses, it may be appropriate to ask for a few volunteers to demonstrate while the others watch. Such an approach makes it clear that not everyone is expected to do the more difficult poses—it may just be fun to try. Some hesitant people may even try the pose when they think everyone is looking at the volunteers.

It is important to offer a good practice for everyone, which means challenging those who love a challenge and creating a safe environment for those who need that support to build confidence. You know you are doing a good job when you get smiles from people of all shapes, sizes, and abilities. And a well-designed and well-executed yoga practice allows you to see these smiles.

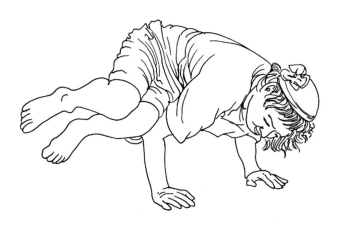

Side Crow

Challenging poses help to build not only strength, but focus and concentration. "If you can calm yourself down in the middle of those poses, you can do it in the middle of the game," said Erroll Simonitisch, a pitcher for the Minnesota Twins. "That's why, before every pitch, you'll see me take a deep breath."[11] So it is good to offer people the opportunity to challenge themselves by developing both their mental and physical skills.

Note: You may work with groups for whom challenging poses are highly inappropriate and would only serve to frustrate people. Some groups need to work well within the safety of a wide comfort zone. It is up to you, as the teacher and guide, to design a practice that suits your group.

Why We Talk About The Breath

The breath should be your teacher.
—T.V.K. Desikachar

We have found that a major appeal of the breath awareness, to people of all ages, is that it is something over which they have control. Stress for many, again of all ages and walks of life, can be rooted in feeling of loss of control. Offering the breath as a healing tool, a calming tool, over which everyone has complete control, is quite appealing.

In yoga we do indeed stretch, but yoga is so much more because of how we work with the breath, or use the breath, to bring ease to both the mind and the body. As Richard Rosen notes in his book, *The Yoga of Breath* (Shambhala, 2002), it is widely accepted that your breath and your state of mind are connected, and that the breath can be used to influence your state of mind. When the body is strong and not tense or fidgety, the mind can find relaxation. But it works both ways—the mind can also bring relaxation to the body. And the mechanism to keep this exchange dynamic is the breath. As A.G. Mohan teaches us, asana practice (poses) should be a harmonious experience, never a struggle.

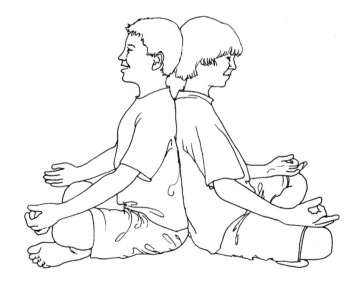

Back to Breathing

"When performed with the graceful orchestration of all its parts, asana can become a music of the body, breath, and mind. Such music moves everything it touches."[12]

And in yoga, it is the act of breathing—how we breathe—and our awareness of this breathing that links the body to the mind. The wonderful thing is that the breath is not something we need to search for to worry about where we are going to store it. As living beings, the breath is already a part of us. But we can change and we can practice how we use this tool. Our common expressions tell us that we already know of the importance of the breath: take a deep breath and count to ten; a breath of fresh air; catch your breath; take your breath away; and breathe easy reflect this awareness of the breath.

Talking about the breath with young people is introducing them to the idea that the breath is something worthy of consideration. So you are giving them a gift—drawing their attention to something they already own. The trick is first to notice it and then to allow it to do its healing, strengthening work. Donna Farhi offers this insight in *The Breathing Book*: "Discovering the naturalness of our breaths has to do with uncovering or removing the obstacles that we have constructed to the breath, both consciously or unconsciously."[13]

For You To Try:

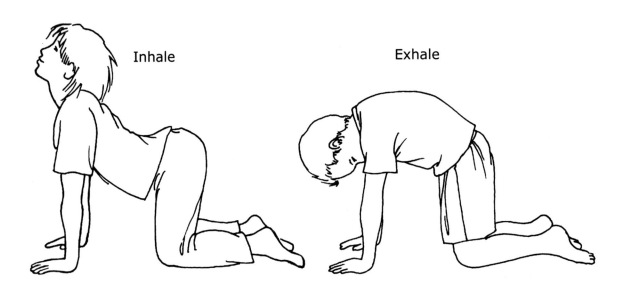

Inhale

Exhale

Cow Pose

Cat Pose

As you consider your own breath and breathing patterns, think about it as a wave and your body movement as a surfer. The wave (breath) begins. Then the surfer (the body moving) begins the ride. The surfer finishes and then the wave is done.[14] A wonderful pose in which to practice this breath/movement idea is cat/cow with the eyes closed. Try it yourself, right now, and see what you think—or rather, try it and see what you *feel*.

Thinking about the breath/movement dance in this way allows us access to the healing benefits of working with the breathing patterns: providing calming and relaxation, lowering blood pressure, lowering heart rate, and decreasing stress hormones to name a few.[15]

How the Body Breathes

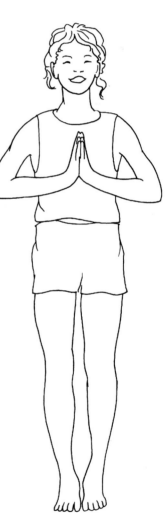

Are you a deep or shallow breather? Do you breathe rapidly, or do you allow your lungs to completely fill with air before you start to exhale? Does it matter? It actually matters to your health and state of mind. Shallow breathing leaves stale air in the bottom part of the lungs, which over time can compromise the health of that lung tissue. Rapid breathing, as when you are upset, causes the heart rate to increase, the blood pressure to rise, and eventually can stress the immune system. When you take a deep breath in and out, you allow for the complete exchange of air in the lungs. The action of the long, slower breath calms the sympathetic (calming) nervous system, contributing to better health. As Lilias Folan notes, the exhale becomes very important because if you are going to fill the vessel, it has to be empty first.

Using the Breath to Draw the Group Back In

1. Yael often uses music in her classes, having found that "listen for the music" creates a quiet room after an interactive (noisy!) sequence. Have people put their hands in *Angeli mudra* (palms to heart center), close their eyes, and listen for the music for about three breaths. The music should not be very loud during a practice, as that in itself can create a distraction.

Mountain Pose

2. Yael developed the following approach one day in a class when a faulty CD player left her with 20 first and second graders and no music. Then she found it worked so well, for some classes she uses no music at all, except for final relaxation. Explain at the start that you will be putting your hands in *Angeli mudra* and listening for your own breath at some times during the practice. Have people close their eyes and listen. You will be pleased at the attention people, even four year-old kids or 15 year-old boys, can give to their own breaths.

3. Another wonderful way to get folks back to their mats after poses that have taken them to the wall or into a big circle, is to say, "Everyone take a deep breath and do not let the breath go until you (and maybe your mat) are back to where we started the class." Yael had kids in a class once that took audible deep breaths and proceeded to zoom around the room until they had to finally let their breaths out, but they were back in their spots. So be prepared to enjoy the kids' creative interpretation of your suggestions. And remember, yoga builds flexibility of the body, but also of the mind!

4. When you are doing a pose (especially a partner pose), explain that everyone will get into the pose and then listen to you. "When everyone has found their boat (or whatever the pose is), let's all take a deep breath in together. Then let the breath out together."

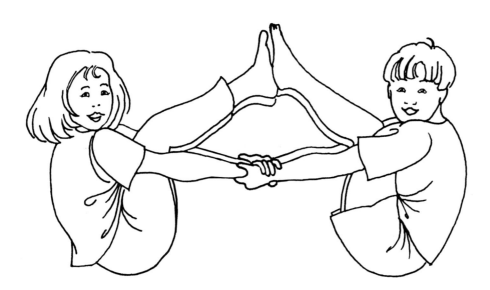

Double Boat

Identify Your Support Team

You may find yourself teaching yoga in a variety of situations. Teaching at a yoga studio or a family program usually does not present the challenge of dealing with disruptive individuals because either the parents are present or the parents have paid for the class.

However, you may find the challenge of dealing with disruptions when teaching in a school or at a summer camp. It is unreasonable to expect a yoga instructor (you) to engage a group in a fun practice and to deal with disruptive, unruly people at the same time. If you are working in a school, perhaps teaching in an after school program, make sure that you know how to address this issue before you begin. Will there be a place to send a person who is not able to participate in yoga today? Will there be camp counselors present as you teach your program? These are reasonable and important questions for you to ask. Teaching yoga to kids and teens is an interactive activity—it will not be quiet. However, an unruly person distracts both you and others from the practice and everyone loses an opportunity to enjoy the benefits of yoga.

We Already Did This Pose . . .

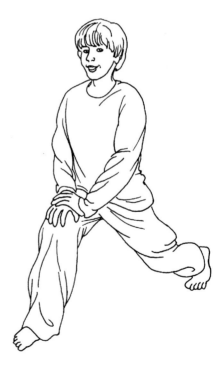

A boy in Yael's class commented, "But we already did this pose." The comment prompted her to explain that while there are traditionally 108,000 yoga poses, we do some poses again because it makes us stronger, allows us to stretch more, and allows us to explore the same poses in a new way. In fact, one classic Hatha yoga text, the Gerandha Samhita, notes that Siva taught 840,000 poses. You will notice that some poses are repeated in the different themes throughout the book, but the approach or sequencing varies. We may come into the pose a different way or talk about different aspects of the pose.

It is important to keep a familiar group of poses so that each class is not all new. People like some familiarity—to be able to find their

Down Dog with only a verbal cue. It is part of making the yoga practice their own. Building that reservoir of familiar poses also allows for more interaction with the group. You can ask such things as, "Which pose lets us balance on one foot?" or "Find a pose that uses only one hand and one foot," or "Let's do some favorites."

In addition, repetition has been found to be a key factor in learning, something studied with great success by the creators of Sesame Street and Blues Clues. Yet, repetition must be paired with some complex ideas to keep the interest level high.[16] So keeping something familiar while introducing new poses and ideas in an interactive format is a key to learning success.

So, yes, we indeed do poses again and again, and hopefully, yet again.

How Should Yoga Feel?

It is important to explain, and to keep mentioning, that yoga is not supposed to hurt. You should feel the sensation of a stretch or a warming in a muscle, which is the muscle working, but you should not feel any pain in the joints or muscles. Some people are schooled to believe that the more it hurts, the better it is for you—a phenomenon easily observed in many health clubs and gyms. Yael's son had a PE teacher who would say, "Stretch until it really hurts. Make it hurt." She did not understand that pain is a signal that something bad thing is happening in the body. So yoga should not cause you pain.

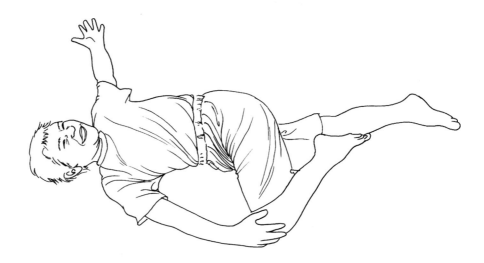

Be Yourself

Do what you can, with what you have, where you are.
—Theodore Roosevelt

When you teach people yoga, you are giving them a great gift—a tool to strengthen both the mind and the body. Students will be looking to you to learn, to help them find ways to have a positive experience. Here is some sage and wonderful advice from Judith Hanson Lasater, author of many books and yoga teacher extraordinaire:

"Be yourself. Remember that you are not only teaching poses, breathing practices,and mediation techniques: you are also sharing skills to help your students live with courage and someday die with grace. Do not worry that you may not know enough. No one does. Be yourself."[17]

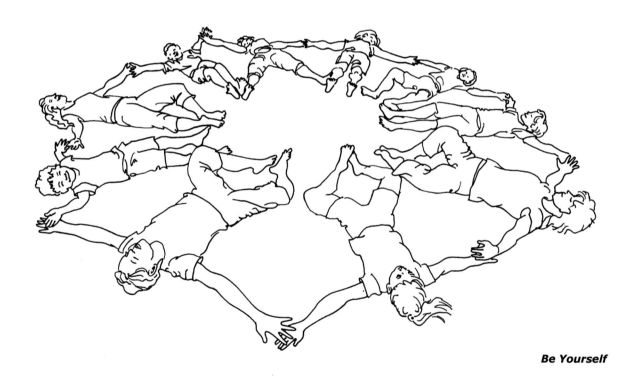

Be Yourself

Namaste!

II. THEMES AND GAMES

Inward calm cannot be maintained
unless physical strength is constantly
and intelligently replenished.
—Buddha

A. Opening Poses

Take the time to at the beginning of any practice to do some opening yoga poses to help people shift gears from their daily activities to settling into a yoga practice. You can find a variety of opening sequences outlined in our first book *Create a Yoga Practice for Kids: Fun, Flexibility, and Focus* (Sunstone, 2006). The following is one sequence followed by some games to make people laugh. Starting with laughter is a way to ensure people are engaged right away and on the track to having a fun practice. Is having fun important? You bet it is. Young people are not going to connect with something that is a chore or done only because you told them it was good for them. So be open to, in fact encourage, the healing powers of laughter, as celebrated in Norman Cousins book *Anatomy of an Illness.*

1. Let's Get Started

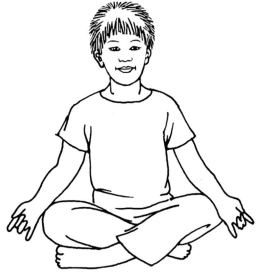

a. Easy Pose *(Sukasana)*

"Let's all take a seat that is easy and comfortable. Press your palms gently against your knees and breathe in, lifting your heart. Let your hands relax in your lap."

Note: A key to a successful class with young people is that it is highly interactive. Introduce yourself, and learn a few names immediately, and try to use a few names throughout the practice. If it is your first class with the group, begin by soliciting ideas about what they think yoga is, and then explain why many athletes like yoga and why you like yoga. (It helps them develop focus, flexibility, relaxation techniques, among other things.) Ask what sports the students do. If it is a large group, ask everyone to

Easy Pose

say together the sport they enjoy doing. Ask them to raise their hands if they know people who do yoga, if they do yoga, or if they know someone who wants to try yoga. It is wonderful for everyone to see the show of hands. Even four year olds like to tell you what they know about yoga! And remember to use this discussion as an opportunity to make immediate connections between you and the class.

b. Breathing

"Now close your eyes and take a deep breath in through you nose. Slowly let go of your breath and begin to let go of anything that has bothered you today—maybe you had the wrong thing for breakfast or you argued with your friend. Take another big breath in and as you breathe out, whisper what bothered you today. (Yael got this idea when kids would do this, unprompted.) Let's take one more breath and slowly let breath out, letting even more go as you push the breath out of your body."

c. Setting intentions

Now we are ready to begin our practice. Put yours hands together at your heart, let your eyes close, and think about what you want to happen during this yoga practice. Do you want to laugh, to have fun, to stretch, to get stronger, to spend time with a friend, or to try something new? Whatever it is, think it in your mind. Then stretch your arms to the sky and open your eyes.

2. Opening Games

People like to play games because games hold their attention and make them laugh and smile. All this lowers stress levels and makes people feel good. Beginning a practice with a game or a silly pose gets people's attention, releases some stress, and brings everyone to a good starting point. Hearing group laughter reinforces that you are in a supportive place.

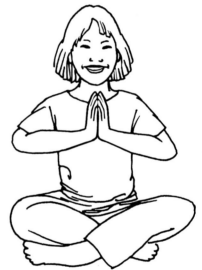

Setting Intentions

a. Make Me Smile

When you smile at life, half the smile is for your face, the other half for somebody else's.
— Tibetan saying

"**Y**oga is actually a science because we are always collecting information—and the fun part is that the information is about us. Instead of learning to ignore things, yoga helps us learn to notice things. Let's be scientists and do an experiment.

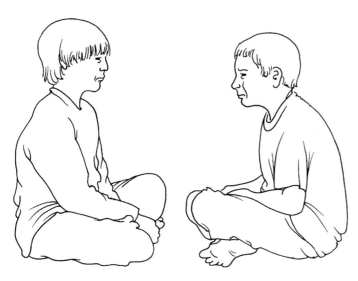

Make Me Smile

You probably have heard that it takes more muscles to frown (43 muscles) than it takes to smile (17 muscles), which means it is easier to smile! Let's see if smiling and frowning can make you feel differently too. Sit and face a friend. First, we are going to make frowning faces. Hold the frown by thinking grumpy and mad thoughts—remember that if we laugh the experiment will not work. So just look into each other's eyes and frown a big frown face. Hold this frown face until I say to stop (30 seconds). Now let your face relax. How do you feel? Now look at your friend, take a deep breath, and make big happy faces with big smiles. Hold your smile until I say to stop (30 seconds). How do you feel now? Next time you see someone, do you think you want to smile or frown at them?"

Note: Science has demonstrated that the human brain prefers a smile over all other facial expressions. The simple act of smiling can affect a person's mood and outlook, and also that of the people around him.[18]

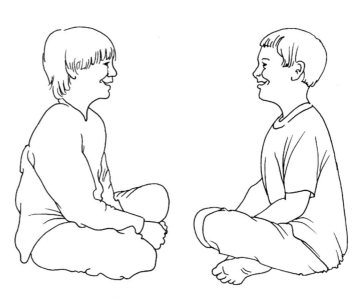

Make Me Frown

b. Keep an Eye Out

"What is a sense that you rely on to figure out where you are? Your eyes collect a lot of visual information. Let's play with that. Stand in Mountain Pose". Do the following sequence, first with your eyes open and then again with your eyes closed.

1) "Breathe in as you lift your toes and shift your weight back onto your heels.

2) On your next breath in, reach your arms toward the sky and lift on to your tip toes. As you breathe out, let your heels come back to your mat.

3) Shift your weight on to your right foot and find some version of Tree Pose. Either rest the left toes on the mat as you lift the left knee, press the sole of the left foot into the calf or the thigh as the standing leg presses back. Do this on both sides.

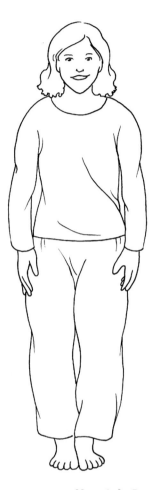

Mountain Pose

Was it easier to keep your balance with your eyes open or closed? Why do you think that it so? Your eyes give your brain important clues about where your body is in space (proprioception *PRO*-pree-o-SEP-shun: the sense of the relative position of your body parts), and what changes your body needs to make so that you do not fall over.

Tree Pose

c. Seasons of Trees*

I think that I shall never see a poem lovely as a tree . . .
—Joyce Kilmer

This sequence is fun to do as the seasons change or as a way to celebrate new spring green colors, fall temperature and color changes, winter shapes, or the cooling summer shade of trees. A balance pose is a wonderful way to get everyone's attention at the start of a practice as they focus on trying to not fall over.

"Let's move through a year of a tree. Imagine your favorite tree that loses its leaves in the winter. You can ask a few people to say their names and favorite tree, another way to learn some names early in the practice. Find a drishti point (focus point at eye level) and stare at it. Shift your weight into your right foot and press the sole of your left foot into your calf or thigh.

1) Winter Tree: (*Vrksasana*) "Put your hands together in palms to heart center. You are a tree in winter, storing food in your roots. Press your foot into the earth and feel those deep, strong roots supporting you. Press your palms together, lift your elbows slightly, and feel your strong trunk."

2) Spring Tree:
"Slowly take a breath in and begin to grow new leaves and branches in the spring. Lift your arms toward the sky as your leaves collect the sunlight to make new food. Feel the sap from your roots start to flow up to your branches."

*Generously offered by Elizabeth Q. Finlinson.

Winter Tree

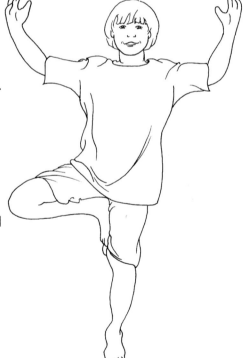

Spring Tree

38

3) Summer Tree:

"Let your arms branch out as your tree fills with leaves, giving shade to everyone who plays under you."

4) Fall Tree:

"As the weather grows colder and the daylight grows shorter, your tree draws energy and food back from the leaves to the roots, so the leaves change color and fall to the ground. Let your arms slowly move down to your side.

Then move back to winter tree, and take two resting breaths with your hand in *Angeli mudra*. Now let's be a different type of tree and do the other side."

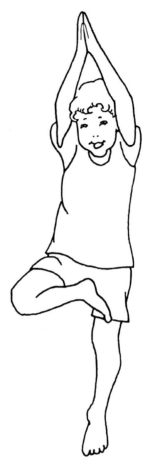

Summer Tree

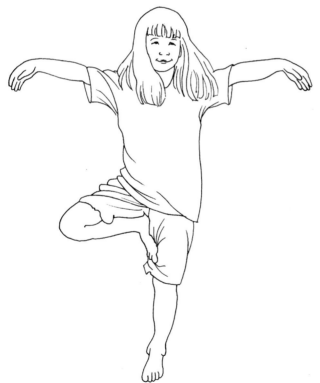

Fall Tree

d. Back to Breathing

Back to Breathing is a pose that can be used in the beginning of practice, in the middle of a practice as a calming pause, or at the end as a way to prepare for final relaxation. It offers people a physical connection to their own breath and to the breath of another person. See where it takes you as you use it in a variety of ways.

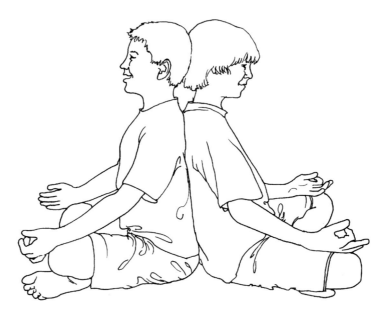

Back to Breathing

"Sit on your mat with your legs folded and your back next to another person. Put your hands on your knees, take a deep breath in, and press your back straight against your friend. Let your hands relax and close your eyes. Let's take four rounds (deep inhale/deep exhale) of breath together. Your eyes are closed so you can really feel the breathing of the other person too."

B. Themes

To teach is to present. And presentation matters. Having spent many years teaching in a wide range of situations, Yael has learned the value of the "hook." It piques the interest, it keeps learning dynamic, and it makes it fun for both the teacher and the student. Keep teaching interesting and fun for you, and your students will take your lead. Themes keep teaching alive. Let them grow as you explore with your students.

1. Stack 'Em Up

Facts About You:

"Guess how many bones you had when you were born? (350). How many do you have now? (206) What happened to your bones? (some fused) Your head has 28 bones. What is the one bone in your head that you can freely move? (mandible, or jawbone).

Part of yoga is about practicing awareness, so this type of question does just that. How come you are not just a pile of the 206 bones in your body?"(Muscles, ligaments and tendons hold the bones together and in place.)

Why Stack the bones? "How can some people in Africa balance and carry very heavy bundles on their heads? If you watch them, they walk very tall and straight, with their bones in good alignment. It takes less energy to carry anything if you walk with good posture. Why do people construct buildings with level foundations and straight beams? In yoga, we try to 'stack the bones' to make sure that we do not pull muscles, stretch out tendons and ligaments, or hurt our joints. It also makes yoga more fun because it takes less energy to stay in a pose."

(1) Invite everyone to slouch forward and try to take a deep breath. Now sit up straight and take a deep breath. Which position allows you to take a deeper breath in? Do you think keeping the spine straight gives our lungs room to fill with breath?

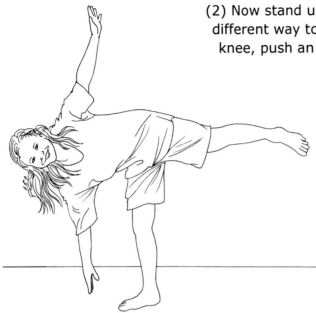

**Stacking the Bones
in Half Moon Pose**

(2) Now stand up and invite everyone to find a different way to lean off center (for example, bend a knee, push an arm out, round the back). Now try to hold that pose for 30 seconds. People will find it difficult and being "out of alignment" causes the muscles to pull and push unevenly. Now stand tall for 30 seconds—feel the difference.

(3) Another way to demonstrate the concept of alignment is to have everyone find a partner. One person stands in a slouch or off center. The other person puts her hands on his shoulders and pushes down—each will see how unstable this position is. Now have the first person stand up straight and tall. Notice if "stacking the bones" or standing in good alignment lends more stability as the other person again presses down on his shoulders. (by permission, from Judith Hanson Lasater's workshops)

a. Mountain Pose (*Tadasana*)

"Let's stack the bones like the beams in a building. Stand at the front of your mat so that the outside of each foot lines up with the outside of each hip. Press your knees forward a little bit, so the knees do not push back (hyperextend). Take a deep breath in and feel the spine lift. Lift your shoulders toward your ears, and as you breathe out, let the shoulder blades roll down your back. Now take a breath in and lift just your toes. Breathe out and let your toes melt back to the earth. You are a rooted mountain. Rock slightly to your right, then slighty to your left. Then come back to 'equal footing', or *Samastithi*, that place when you feel your bones stacked over your feet."

Benefits: Mountain Pose provides the opportunity to practice standing in good alignment, a practice that helps prevent the many back problems associated with poor posture or slouching.

**Stacking the Bones
in Mountain**

b. Rooster Pose

"Can we keep our stacked bones if we shift our weight forward? As you take a deep breath in, lift your heels and sweep your arms to the sky. Does this feel differently than Mountain Pose? Breathe out and lower your heels and your palms to heart center. Let's do this several more times. The pose is called Rooster Pose, so you can make the sound of a rooster as you lift up. But stop crowing when your heels hit the ground, because then you are back to being a strong, quiet mountain."

Challenge: Do this pose 10 times, sweeping the arms to the sky and 10 times with the hands in palms to heart center.

Benefits: Rooster Pose builds strength in the calf muscles, stretches the feet and ankles, and develops focus and concentration.

c. Side Plank Pose (Vasisthasana)

"We have 30 bones in each of our arms and legs, for a grand total of how many bones? Let's stack our bones another way. Find your Down Dog Pose. Drop your right knee to the mat, roll onto the inside of your left foot, and shift your weight onto your right hand. Look to see that your foot, knee, and hand are lined up. Now lift your hips and reach your left arm to the sky. Inhale tall as you stack your 60 arm bones in one tall stack. Take two breaths and then come out of the pose. Let's do it once more on this side. Then find your way back into Down Dog and do Side Plank on the left side.

Challenge: Extend the right leg and rest on the outside of the right foot, then stack the inside of left foot on top on it. Lift the hips. Lift the left leg and take three breaths, extending the top arm past the ear.

Benefits: Side Plank builds core strength and concentration. It also strengthens the arms and back.

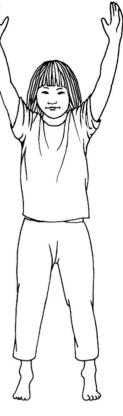

Rooster

Side Plank

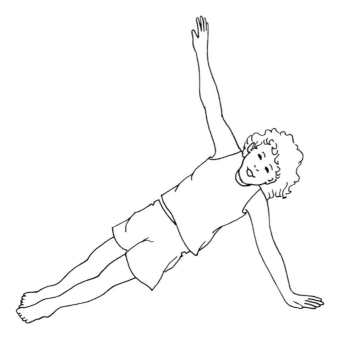

Side Plank Challenge

d. Lifted-Leg Side Plank

"Let's try a different version of Side Plank. Find Down Dog Pose. Then move into Side Plank with your right knee on the mat. What happens if you tip your stacked bones slightly forward? Find your perfect alignment again and take two more breaths. Come out of the pose and do it one more time on this side. Then do the other side, to give your muscles an equal chance to get strong and stretched."

Challenge: Bend your raised left leg and reach back with your left hand and grab the left ankle. Open the heart as you find your backbend. For even more of a challenge, straighten the right leg so you are resting on the outside of the right foot. Then lift the left leg, grasp the ankle, and find your backbend.

Benefits: The pose allows people to explore their balance points and build core and leg strength.

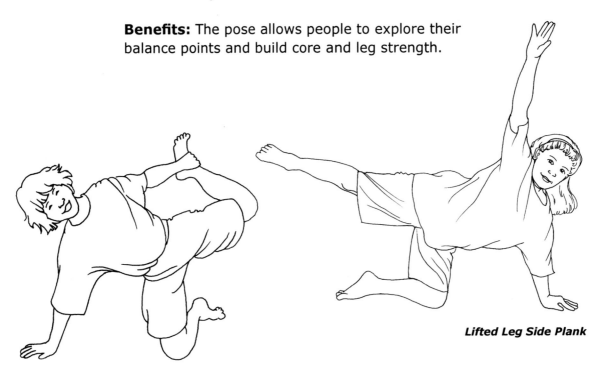

*Side balance
Challenge 2*

Lifted Leg Side Plank

e. Half Moon at the Wall (Ardha Chandrasana)

"Did you know that yoga is a science? Yoga is about collecting information about yourself. So let's be scientists. We are going to do a pose on the mat, and then move to a wall to do the same pose. It is an experiment to see which way you think is easier.

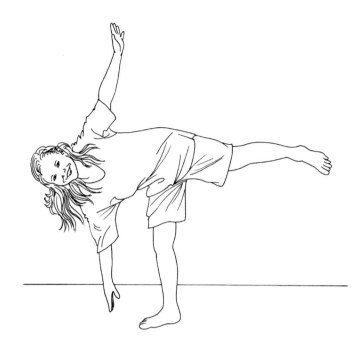

Half Moon

1) Half Moon on the Mat
Stand in Mountain Pose. Step the left foot back. Check to see that your right front foot is parallel to the mat because this gives you the most stability in the pose. Now bend the front knee and slowly shift your weight forward over the front foot. Move forward until your right hand is resting on the floor. Turn your chest open so it shines on the wall, just like the light shining from the moon. Do you feel stable and strong? Do you think your bones are stacked tall or are some leaning over?

2) Half Moon at the Wall
Now we are going to do the same pose at the wall. You do not need your mats. Stand with your right foot parallel to the wall, about five inches away. Remember not to move that front foot—wiggle your ears or your eyelashes to keep your balance, but do not move the foot! Lean your whole body against the wall and slowly let the right hand drop toward the floor as you lift the left leg. Your hand might not reach the floor, and that is fine. Hold the pose for three breaths. Then do the other side. Which Half Moon felt stronger? Which was easier to hold? We can really stack the bones when we lean against the wall."

Challenge: From Half Moon on the mat, reach around with the left hand and grasp the left ankle. Explore whatever backbend you find here.

Benefits: This pose strengthens the gluteus muscles, the core stabilizing muscles, and the standing leg. It also is a confidence-building pose as the body is open but feels strong at the same time.

f. Reverse Handstand at the Wall
(Parivritta Adho Mukha Vrksasana)

"Take your mats to the wall. Sit against the wall and press your heels into the mat. That is the point where you are going to place your palms. Do a short Down Dog against the wall, then walk one leg up the wall and then the other."

Challenge: Walk the feet down so your shoulders are over your hands and your body is at a 90 degree bend. Take three breaths here and then walk your legs back up the wall.

Benefits: The inversion stimulates the lymph circulation (it only moves

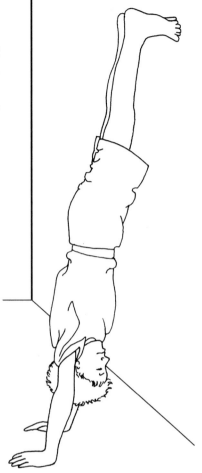

Reverse Half Handstand

when you do)—the lymphatic fluids carry the body's immune cells: white blood cells, macrophages, T-cells are some examples. If you do not move, it's like an army trying to fight a battle but staying in the barracks!

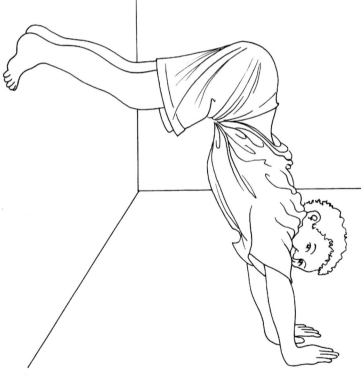

Reverse Half Handstand

2. Muscle Magic

Facts About You:

"What moves the bones? Muscles do. You have three kinds of muscles: skeletal, smooth, and cardiac. The skeletal muscles move the bones. Skeletal muscles attach to the bones by tendons. We can control these muscles by thinking. Can you wave your little finger? Can you move your middle finger and ring finger apart? You did that by thinking about it.

But muscles have help holding up the bones. Ligaments and tendons help keep bones in place. Ligaments connect bone to bone, while tendons connect bones to muscles. Tendons and ligaments have a limited blood supply, so they take a longer time to heal than muscles do. You do not want to overstretch muscles, tendons or ligaments. So if something hurts, stop doing it!"

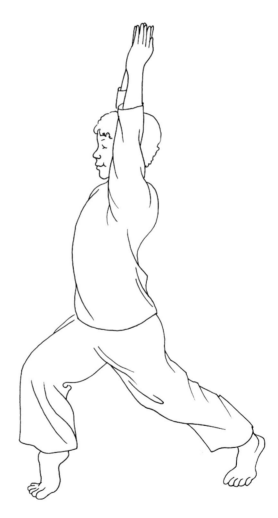

"There are two groups of muscles that work even without our telling them to: smooth muscles, like the muscles in the stomach and intestines, and the cardiac muscles in the heart. That is a good thing or we would have to stay awake at night to tell our heart to beat and our stomachs to digest dinner.

We always have the same number of muscle fibers in our body, although it is a different number for each person. When we exercise the muscles we do have, they get stronger and bigger. Let's do some poses to build our skeletal muscles."

Muscles Lifting the Bones

a. Chair Pose Flow *(Utkatansa)*

"Think about the helium balloons you might see at a birthday party. On a big breath in, lift your arms to the sky in tall mountain pose. As you breathe out, spread your arms like wings and gently float toward the floor as you come up on your toes. Take two breaths here. Then give yourself a hug and be a balloon at rest. What color balloon are you? Now picture that helium balloon as you fill your chest with breath and lift back up—you are so light, just like the balloon. Stretch to the sky in tall mountain pose. Do this once more."

Floating

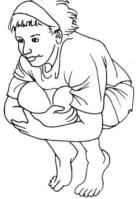

Balloon Landing

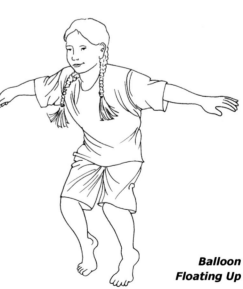

Challenge: Do this pose in slow motion. The more slowly you move, the stronger your muscles will get. Now do it in even slower motion!

Balloon Floating Up

48

Benefits: This flow strengthens the thigh muscles (the quadriceps), and the calf muscles. It also gives people the opportunity to practice moving with the breath as they rise on the inhale and release down, with the breath, on the exhale. In addition, it offers people the time to practice visualization, a powerful healing and strengthening tool.

b. Warrior 1 *(Virabhadrasana 1)*: **Flow and Variation**

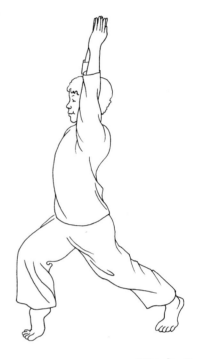

"There are three yoga poses that make you feel strong because they build strength in your body and in your mind. You need strong muscles to hold a warrior pose. You also need to keep your focus or pay attention to what your body is doing, which makes your mind strong. Let's do all three Warrior poses. You decide which one you think makes you grow the strongest.

Find Mountain Pose at the front of your mat. Step your left foot back and balance on your toes (or you can spin the back foot flat onto the mat, the more challenging way). As if you have a light in your belly button, shine it forward. Take a breath in and lift your arms to the sky. As you release your breath, bend the front leg and melt down. Be strong by lifting the arms higher toward the sky. Hold this pose for three breaths. Then step back into Mountain Pose and do the other side."

Warrior 1

Variation: Create a flow as you inhale up to straighten the leg and put the hands to heart center in *Angeli mudra*. Then exhale as you lift the arms to the sky and bend the front knee. Create this flow by using the breathing in and breathing out to guide the body movement. Do the flow three times to build strength.

Challenge: Do reverse *Angeli mudra* while in Warrior 1. Place your palms to heart center behind your back and then exhale as you lean forward over your front leg. You can also interlace your fingers behind your back and lift them. Bend forward over the front leg as you breathe out.

For another challenge, try to switch sides by jumping! So, jump the right foot back while you bring the left foot forward. This challenge always brings giggles.

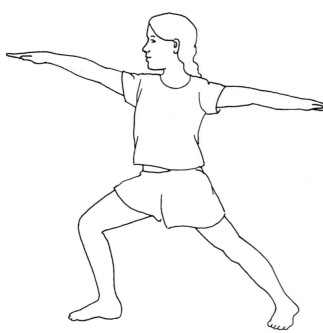

Warrior 2

c. Warrior 2 (*Virabhadrasana*): **Flow and Variation**

Find Mountain Pose at the front of your mat. Step your left foot back. Then check to see that the back of your foot is parallel to the back of the mat. The light in your belly button is shining toward the left side of the room. Take a breath in and lift your arms out like a "T", and as you breathe out, bend the front leg. Hold for three breaths, step the foot forward into Mountain Pose and repeat on the other side.

Variation: Create a flow to build muscle strength as you breathe in and release the arms to your side and straighten the front leg, and then breathe out as you bend the front knee, lift the arms, and find the pose. Do the flow three times.

Challenge: From Warrior 2, put your left hand on your left hip, turn your right palm to the sky, and sweep the right hand toward the back, feeling that front body stretch and the legs strengthen. Exhale back into Warrior 2 for three breaths. Then do the other side.

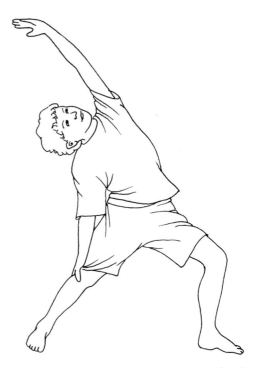

Reverse Warrior 2

d. Warrior 3 (*Virabhadrasana 3*): **Flow and Variation**

"Find Mountain Pose. Take a breath in and lift your arms to the sky. As you breathe out, reach your spine forward as you stretch your arms and lift your back leg. Remember, this is your pose, so only lift the leg as high as you can and still feel strong. You are strengthening the largest muscle in your body, the gluteus maximus. Feel the strength in your body and in your mind—you need a strong mind to hold this pose."

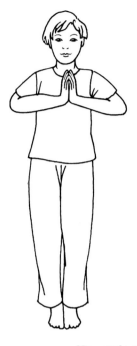

Mountain Pose

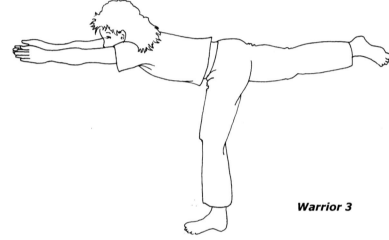

Warrior 3

Variation: Create a flow by lifting the arms and bringing the extended leg forward to Tree Pose.

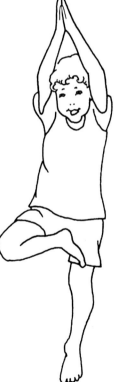

Tree Pose

Challenge: Begin in Mountain Pose. Step back into Warrior 1. Then spin your back heel and move into Warrior 2. Take a deep breath in and exhale forward into Warrior 3. Then finish the flow as you bend your front leg and step back to "land the lunge". Can you do it without looking back? That is the challenge! Repeat on the other side

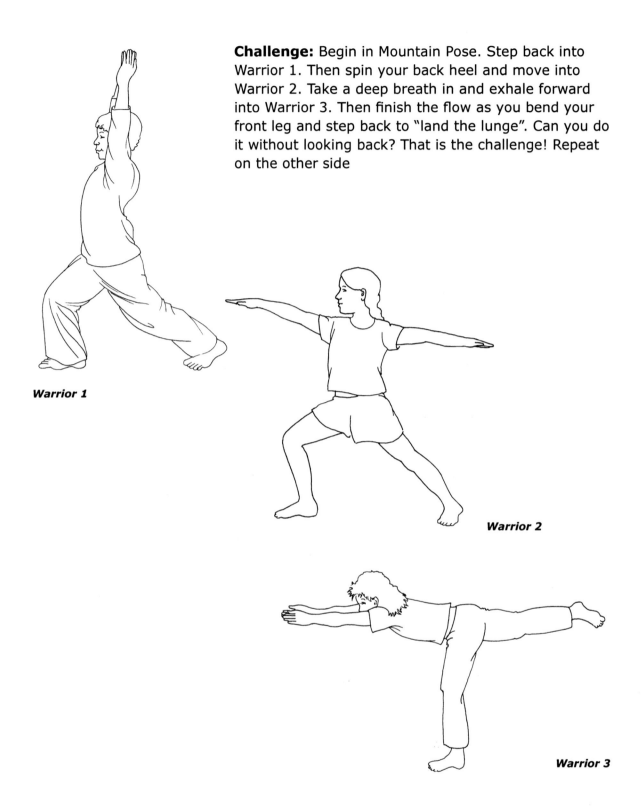

Warrior 1

Warrior 2

Warrior 3

Benefits: The Warrior series builds strength in the legs, core, and back. The flow variation builds stamina and deepens the awareness of the connection between the breath and movement.

e. Dolphin

"Dolphins are very strong swimmers. Picture a graceful dolphin jumping out of the water with its back arching up. Keep that image of a powerful jump that lifts as you lift your hips toward the sky into Down Dog. Then release your elbows down so they rest under your shoulders on the mat. (Remember stacking the bones? This alignment gives you more strength). Lift your hips another inch as you picture that dolphin arching its back toward the sun. Take three breaths here. Then sit back on your feet and lift your arms toward the sky. As you exhale, come back into dolphin pose, keeping the image of that strong dolphin in your mind as you close your eyes, lift, and breathe."

"Dolphins will help an injured member of their group, or pod, to the surface of the water so it can breathe. Maybe you need to be strong to help a friend or someone in your family."

Challenge: Walk the feet closer to the front of the mat. This pose is a preparation for headstand as it builds strong core muscles.

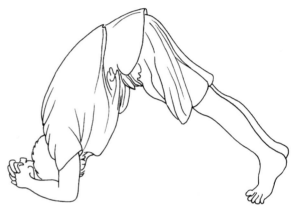

Dolphin

Benefits: The pose builds arm and core strength. The imagining exercise also helps to develops the skill of visualization, a powerful tool in physical development and healing. In addition, the inversion (hips above the head) stimulates the flow of lymph (immune system) in the body.

3. Step It Up: All About Feet

*A journey of a thousand miles
begins with a single step.
—Lao-tzu*

Feet make a fun theme because there is so much bouncing and balancing and motion to explore. Many of us are not as nice to our feet as we should be. After all, they do carry us where we need to go, usually not complaining until we stuff them into odd-shaped footwear. If we do not heed their complaints, or fail to process the information our bodies are sending us, the signals grow louder until our feet really hurt. Foot problems can grow into hip issues, back issues and even shoulder problems—the foot bone is indeed connected to the leg bone and so on. Play with the firm foundation offered by the feet.

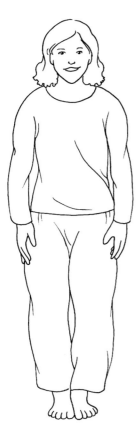

Facts About You:

"Each foot has 26 bones, so one quarter of all the bones in your body are in your feet! Each foot and ankle has more than 100 muscles, tendons (fibrous tissues that connect muscles to bones), and ligaments (fibrous tissues that connect bones to other bones)."

a. Mountain Pose *(Tadasana)* or *(Samastithi)*(sam is TEE' ta he)(Equal Standing)

Note: Mountain Pose is classically done with the feet together, while in *Samstithi*, the feet are hip width apart, allowing for equal standing.

"Stand tall at the front of your mat with the outside of your feet lined up with the outside of your hips ("Equal Standing). Shift your weight to your heels (the calcaneum bones) as you lift your toes. As you breathe out again, come forward on your toes. Breathe in and lower down, pressing your feet into the mat. Now lean a little to the right, then a little to the left. Come back to center and put your hands in palms to heart center. Do your feet help you balance?"

Mountain Pose

Challenge: Lift your arms to the sky, interlace your fingers, and exhale forward into Warrior 3. Feel how the standing foot connects more firmly to the earth. Now bend the front knee and step the raised leg back into a lunge. Now put your weight on your front foot as you glide forward into Warrior 3. To challenge yourself one more time, end the flow by finding your in Tree Pose.

Benefits: Finding good posture in Mountain Pose allows the chest to open, giving more room in the thoracic cavity for the heart and the lungs to function properly. The challenge flow builds stamina, balance, and core strength.

b. Rooster

"Has anyone ever known a rooster? What would be a good way to stretch out all the muscles and make some space in all those 33 joints in each foot? See if you can feel this stretch in your feet. Take a deep breath in, sweep your arms to the sky and come up on your toes. Breathe out as you come down. Let's do this ten times. Did you know that your big toe has two bones, but all the other toes have three bones? Can you stay up on your toes for two full breaths? Come back to Mountain Pose, hands in *Angeli mudra*, and close your eyes. Notice how your feet feel.

How are the muscles in your feet connected to your back? Let's do four more Roosters and see if we feel anything in our backs."

Benefits: Rooster Pose draws awareness to the feet and offers the opportunity to practice balance, to stretch out the muscles and connective tissue on the bottoms of the feet, stretch and strengthen the toe and ankle muscles, and practice moving with the breath. This simple up/down motion provides an opportunity to coordinate the breath with the movement, a key part of any yoga practice.

Rooster

c. **Down Dog** (*Adho Mukha Savanasana*)

"Plant your hands and your feet on the mat, making your body into a big 'V' shape. Lift up onto your toes and stretch your hips toward the sky. Now pedal your feet, as if you are on a bike—lift one heel and then the other. Pay attention to the feet and see how many different ways you can rest on them. Did you roll to the outside edge of one and the inside edge of the other? What else can you do to stretch the feet?"

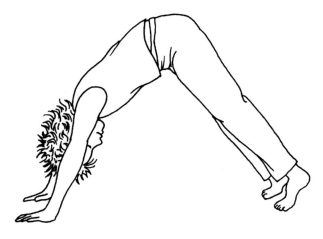

Down Dog

Variation: From Down Dog, roll onto the outside edge of the right foot and the inside edge of the left foot. Go back into Down Dog and switch sides. Find your Down Dog once again. Roll over the tops of your toes, for a toe massage, and come into Up Dog. As you breathe out, roll over the tops of your toes again to come into Down Dog.

Challenge: From the pose, lift the right leg to the sky. Make circles with your feet and toes, three times in one direction, three times in the other. Then switch legs. Find your Down Dog again, and lift the right leg. Bend the right knee and drop the leg open to the left.

Benefits: Down Dog strengthens the arms and back while stretching the legs. As a full body stretch, the pose is relaxing too. Looking at the world from a different angle allows for a possible change in perspective. Down Dog can be like a whole yoga practice in itself. Take time to play with it.

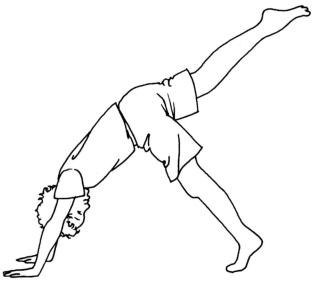

Raised Mountain

d. Toe Lunge

"Stand in Mountain Pose and step the left foot to the back of your mat, staying up on your toes. Lift the back heel high off the ground. Now can you lift the front heel up and balance on both your front and back toes (or lift one heel and then set it down before you lift the other)? To find a wonderful foot massage, breathe in and lift the front heel, then breathe out and press the front foot into the mat. Try this massage for five wonderful breaths. Then step the left foot up to Mountain Pose, breathe your hands to the sky as you stretch to a tall mountain. Then do the other side."

Variation: Bend the front knee as you exhale and lift the front heel. As you take a deep breath in, lift the arms to the sky, straighten the front leg and then come up on all ten toes. Exhale and release the feet to the mat and bend the front leg, coming up on all ten toes again. Invite people to play with the different patterns of breathing and lifting the heels.

Benefits: This pose stretches the toes and strengthens the legs muscles. It also allows people to explore and to strengthen their balance.

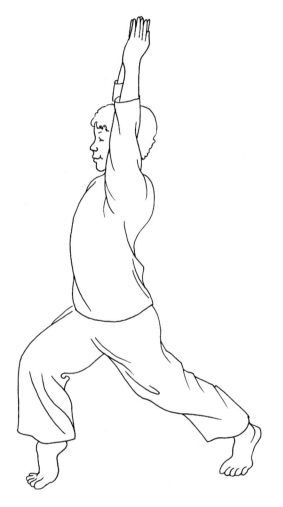

Toe Lunge

e. Warrior 3 *(Virabhadrasana 3)* **to a Lunge** *(Anjaneyasana)*

"Let's see how our feet support us. Feel your feet give you firm support in Mountain Pose, then take a deep breath in and lift the left leg toward the back and lift your hands to the sky. As you breathe out, bend forward into Warrior 3. You are standing on only one foot. Let's use the other foot now by bending the front knee and kicking that left leg back to a lunge. If you like, try lifting up on to the toes, as you just did in the last pose. Find Mountain Pose and do the other side."

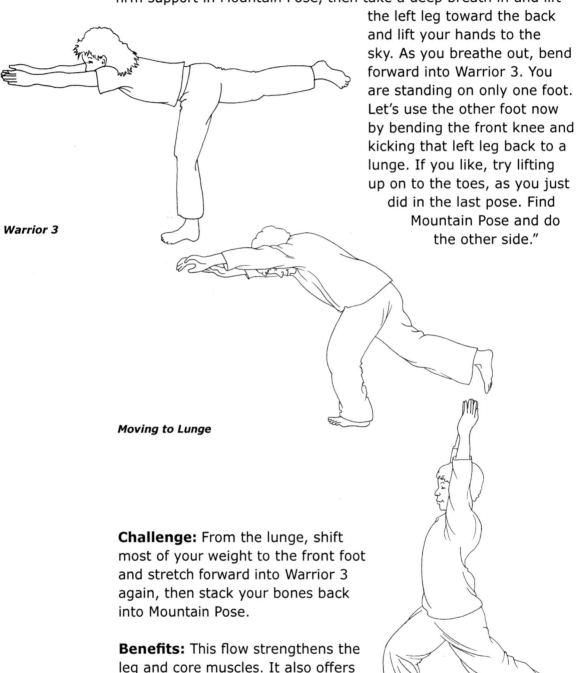

Warrior 3

Moving to Lunge

Challenge: From the lunge, shift most of your weight to the front foot and stretch forward into Warrior 3 again, then stack your bones back into Mountain Pose.

Benefits: This flow strengthens the leg and core muscles. It also offers a chance to practice balance while focusing on the way the feet contact the earth.

Lunge

f. Tree Pose *(Vrksasana)*

"From Mountain Pose, find a drishti point—something at eye level on which you can fix your gaze. Shift your weight into your right foot and really press down through the whole foot as you lift your left leg into Tree Pose. Can you grow as you lift onto your tiptoes? Take two breaths and do the other side."

Challenge: From Tree Pose, take a deep breath in and stretch out into Warrior 3. Hold it for two breaths and stretch back into a lunge. For even more of a challenge, shift forward again into Warrior 3. Can you breathe in and lift the toes and let the breath go as you bring the feet to the floor?

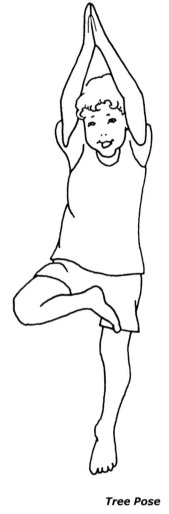

Benefits: Tree Pose strengthens the muscles and the vasculature (arteries, veins and capillaries) in the standing leg.

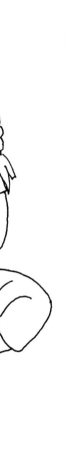

Tree Pose

Tree Pose

g. Thunderbolt *(Vajrasana)*

"Usually we stand on our feet. How would it look if we used are feet as a seat cushion? Sit back on your feet, the tops of the feet resting on the floor. Press your palms against your knees as you take a big breath in and lift the heart. Keep that lift as you breathe out. Let's hold this pose for three breaths. How else can we sit on our feet? Curl your toes under and sit back. Does this stretch feel different? Stay here for three breaths."

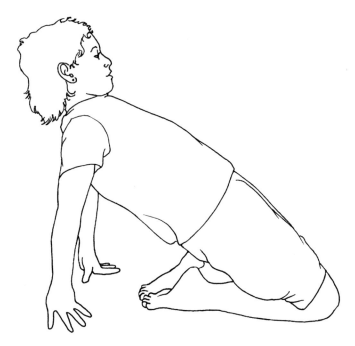

Thunderbolt

Challenge: Put your palms on the floor behind you under your shoulders and lift your hips toward the sky.

Benefits: This pose stretches out the muscles and the bottom of the feet and the quadriceps.

4. Celebrate the Cerebellum: Balance

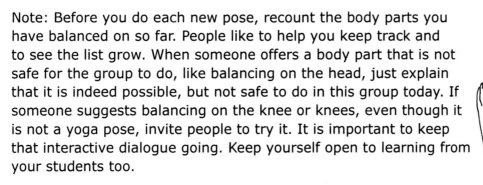

Life is like riding a bicycle.
To keep your balance you must keep moving.
—Albert Einstein

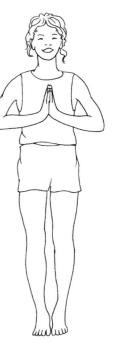

Kids of all ages like balance poses because they are a challenge, they allow the mind to clear of clutter (too many thoughts), and they are entertaining to try and to watch others try. People also like to see how quickly they progress from one class to next.

Facts About You:
"The cerebellum (sarah BELL um) is called the little brain. It is located at the base of the brain stem. Its function is to coordinate all muscles when you move, like when you walk, talk, and balance. It also controls your fine motor skills. Let's give our cerebellum something to think about!

Let's guess how many body parts we can balance on. Can you balance on your nose? Your toes? Your elbows? Let's keep track as we go and see if we guessed them all."

Mountain Pose

Note: Before you do each new pose, recount the body parts you have balanced on so far. People like to help you keep track and to see the list grow. When someone offers a body part that is not safe for the group to do, like balancing on the head, just explain that it is indeed possible, but not safe to do in this group today. If someone suggests balancing on the knee or knees, even though it is not a yoga pose, invite people to try it. It is important to keep that interactive dialogue going. Keep yourself open to learning from your students too.

a. Mountain Pose *(Tadasana)*

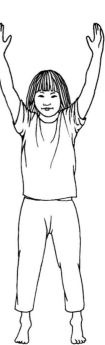

"Stand like a mountain and then look down at your feet. Not very much of you is touching the earth, is it? But you are balancing just fine. Now close your eyes. Do you notice a change in your balance?"

Variation: Can you balance on just your toes? Come up into Rooster Pose and stay here for three breaths.

Benefits: Mountain Pose allows a person to explore how it feels to stand straight and tall with a firm foundation on the earth. Such alignment is important for good posture, which is so important in protecting the back from possible strains and injuries.

Rooster Pose

b. Tree Pose *(Vrksasana)* and Variations

"How many years have you been practicing balancing on two feet? So let's try one foot. Stare at a point right in front of you to 'fix your gaze.' Shift your weight into your right foot and lift your left knee up slowly. Then turn the knee toward the side of the room. Find the tree that is right for you. Maybe your left toe is still on the ground, maybe the bottom of your left foot is pressing into your right calf, and maybe your left foot is pressing into your right thigh. Trees come in all shapes and sizes! Think about your tree roots going deep into the earth. Think about stretching your branches toward the sky so your leaves get a lot of sunlight. Now stand on two feet before you try to be a tree on the other side."

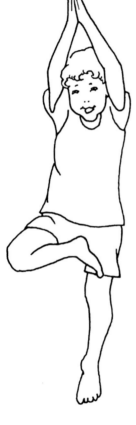

Variation: Stand on the right foot and cross the left ankle over the top of the right knee. Take a deep breath in and as you breathe out, melt down as you sit back into Bush Pose.

Challenge: For a deeper challenge, fold forward from Bush Pose and touch your fingertips on the floor. You can also fold forward and place the palms on the floor, resting your front shin on your upper arms as you press forward into an arm balance. To come out of the pose, slowly lift and grow into Tree Pose.

Benefits: Tree Pose builds focus, concentration and balance. It also gives an opportunity to practice visualization as people imagine the tree roots giving them stability or connection with the Earth. Invite the students to imagine their favorite type of tree and where it is growing. Bush Pose is a great way to stretch the hips muscles and strengthen the standing leg.

Tree Pose

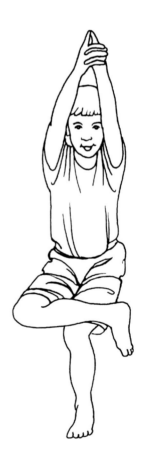

Bush Pose

c. Crow (or Crane) (*Bakasana*)

"Who likes to laugh? Okay, get ready to laugh. Look at your hands and move the fingers all around. How many bones do you think are in each hand? (27 bones) Squat down and put your hands, fingers spread like starfish rays, on the mat. Press your knees together as you push your elbows apart. Feel how that makes the muscles in your belly work!

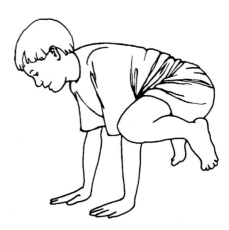

Crow Pose 1

Those are the muscles that will help to lift you in this balance. Lean forward on your starfish hands. Lift one foot, perhaps resting only the big toe on the earth, then lift the other. Remember, you can keep both feet on the floor if that is your Crow."

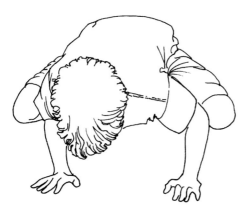

Variation:
Crow Pose 2

Variation: You can also rest your thighs on the tops of your arms (triceps). For some people, this is easier. So offer it as a variation, or, from a squatting position, tuck your arms inside your legs and balance on your hands in crane pose.

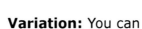
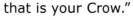

Challenge: Side Crow (*Parsva Bakasana*)
From a squat, twist around to the left side, bringing the top of your right arm over the outside of your left thigh. Plant both palms on the left side on the floor, in line with your leg. Slowly tip to the left, engaging your core muscles as you lift onto your right arm.

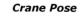

Crane Pose

Benefits: This pose always gets a lot of laughs, which is a great stress release. It builds confidence and the sense of being in a safe environment to try new things.

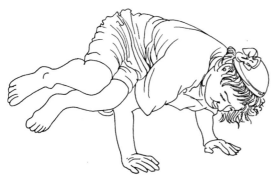
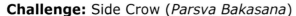

Side Crow

d. Help Name This Side Balance

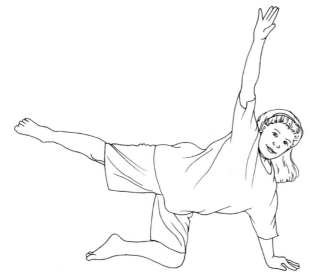

Name This Pose!

"This pose needs a name, so let's try to find a name for it. Find your Down Dog first. Move around and give one bark like your favorite dog. Then drop your right knee and roll onto the inside of your left foot so that your right hand and right knee are in a line. Let's lift the left leg, but keep your balance. The challenge is to reach around and grasp your left ankle with your left hand in side balance. On what are we balancing?

Challenge: Do the same pose, but do not drop the right knee. Instead, roll onto the outside of the right foot into Side Plank. Can you now lift the left leg and then reach back and grasp the left ankle with the left hand?

Remember, the challenge poses are just for fun and to keep everyone's interest. But, you may have a group where challenge poses are not at all appropriate.

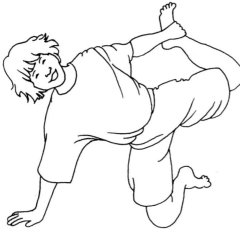

Side Balance

Benefits: Having the students name a pose involves them in the practice, especially if you will be meeting with them again. The side balance pose builds focus, as the core and the gluteus muscles strengthen to give stability to the pose.

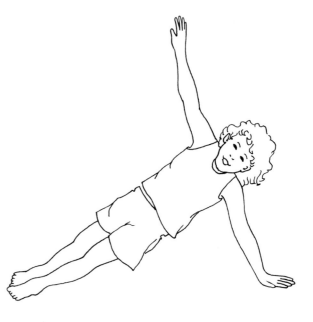

Side Plank

e. One-Sided Balance

"Can you think of another way to balance on one hand and the knee and foot? Show me your ideas. Come to a Flatback. First extend out the right hand and lift the left leg. Take a deep breath in and slowly let your breath out. We just balanced on the opposite hand and leg. Now come back to Flatback. Repeat on the other side."

Variation: Open the raised arm and leg out to the side and take a breath.

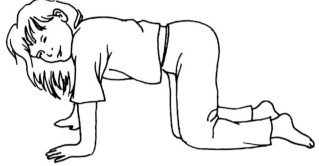

Flatback

Challenge: From Flatback, take a breath in and lift the right arm and then lift the right leg! Play with this for a few breaths and see what happens. Come back to Flatback and feel how stable your body feels. Now try the other side.

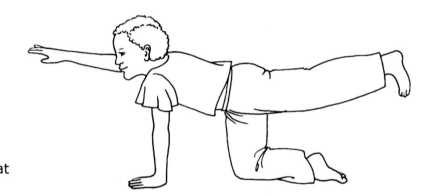

Flatback Balance

Benefits: A major benefit of this pose is that is encourages laughter. Suggest that people can laugh at themselves, at you, or at the guy next to them—just have some fun with it. Laughter decreases stress hormones, strengthens the immune system and makes people enjoy yoga. If they don't have fun, they will not want to do yoga. Then they will miss all the great benefits. And of course, the pose builds balance and core strength too.

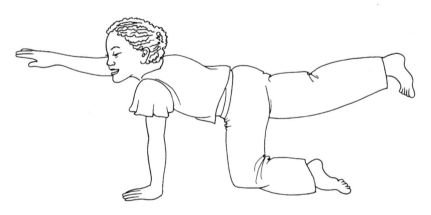

Same Side Flatback Balance

f. Boat Pose

"Can you balance on something you usually do not look at very much on yourself? Well, you probably do not spend a lot of time looking at your bum! Show me how you think it might look to balance on your bum. You can keep your knees bent or you can wrap your arms around the backs of your thighs. Where is your boat going? Are you on the ocean or in a lake? When everyone is in their boat, let's all take a breath in together, and then breathe out together."

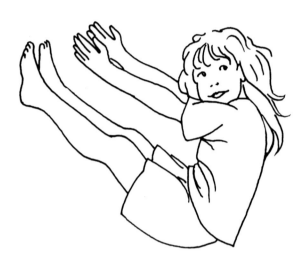

Boat Pose

Variation: Straighten your legs as you lift them and lift your arms straight in front of you. Can you grasp your ankles and make the boat into a very deep "V" bottomed boat? Now press the soles of your feet together and hold your ankles, like a lifting butterfly.

Challenge: Grab your feet (or ankles or calves) and lift your legs up straight to make yourself into a "V". You can then open your legs out to the sides. Play with your balance here. Keep a slight rounding in your back because it makes it harder to engage your core muscles if you bend back. You an also grasp your feet and open your legs into a wide 'V' shape. If someone rolls back, say, "What a wonderful way to massage your spine!"

Benefits: Boat Pose builds core strength, works the quadriceps, and develops focus and concentration. It also makes people laugh, always a benefit to the system.

g. Swimmer Pose

"Now how would you look balancing on the opposite body part? Lie on your belly and take a deep breath in as you lift your arms and your legs off the mat."

Note: It is more accurate to say, "Lie on your belly (or tummy)," instead of saying stomach, as the stomach is an organ. We are trying to engage the abdominal muscles,

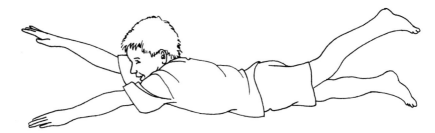

Swimmer Pose 1

which strengthen our poses and allow us to deepen our exhalation. To locate the belly area, have people place a thumb on the navel, with the hand below that. The area under the hand is the belly!

Variation: Extend the right arm forward and lift the left leg. Hold for two breaths and then switch sides. You an also reach around and grab your left ankle with your right hand.

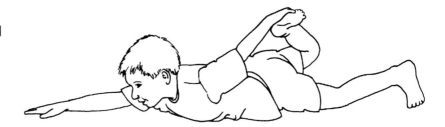

Swimmer Pose 2

Challenge: Reach around and grab your ankles and on a big breath in, lift up into Bow Pose. Feel how you are balancing on your belly as you lift higher using your breath to fill your bow. After two breaths, release down and rest for two breaths. Now try it again since your muscles are all warmed and ready to go.

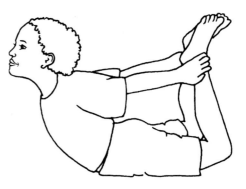

Bow Pose

Benefits: Swimmer poses stretch out the thighs (quadriceps) and the front hip flexors, strengthen the lower back, and stretch the shoulders.

h. Warrior 3 and Standing Bow

The following set of poses can be done at a wall. Warrior 3 and Standing Bow can be done on a mat, but it may be easier for some people to lean one palm against a wall (or they can balance by resting a hand a partner's shoulder). It depends on the group, so as with doing your own yoga practice, make the necessary adjustments to make it work for you.

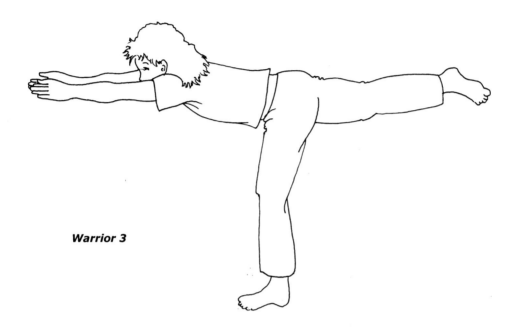

Warrior 3

"Let's get back to balancing on one foot. Let's be a strong warrior, using our strong minds to help our bodies stand in a powerful balance. Remember, not all warriors look the same, so I invite you to be the warrior that is right for you. Take a deep breath in and lift your arms to the sky. As you breathe out, bend forward and begin to move the left foot toward the back of the room. If the toes rest on the mat, that is fine. Be your own warrior.

Make your hips flat like a table, so if I put a glass of lemonade on your hips it would not fall off. Be strong in your warrior for two or three breaths and then find Mountain Pose. Pause for a moment with your eyes closed and whisper why you need to be strong in your body or in your thinking. Take a breath in and open your eyes. Now balance on the other foot to find your Warrior 3 on the left leg."

Variation: Stand in Crescent Moon Pose. Take a breath in and bend your arms to the right, lifting your left leg off the mat toward the left. Then exhale around and forward to Warrior 3.

Challenge: Standing Bow

"You are getting really good at balancing on one leg. Who is ready to do a very challenging balance? The trick to this pose is to keep your standing foot lined up with the outside edge of your mat and not to let it wiggle around. So to keep your balance, you can wiggle your ears, your fingers, your nose, or even your eyelashes, but do not move that foot. (This stance provides the most stable alignment because the top of the femur has the most surface contact with the pelvis.) From Warrior 3, lift up and then reach around and grab your left ankle with your left hand. Reach your right arm out about 45 degrees as you kick you leg up a bit more!"

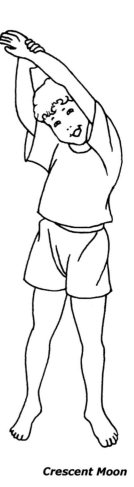

Crescent Moon

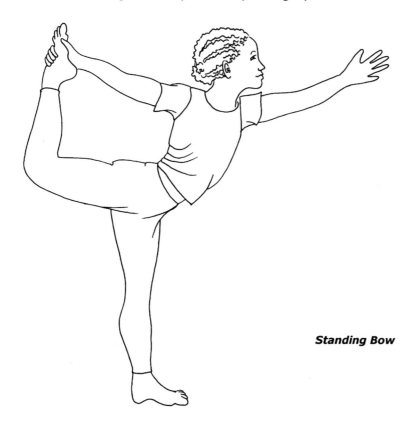

Standing Bow

Benefits: Using a wall or a friend's shoulder to bring stability to a pose lets people know it is good to find support when needed. It helps to strengthen the proper muscles for the pose and decreases stress on the joints.

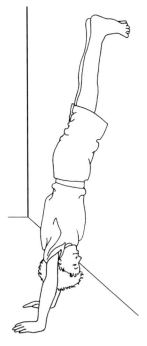

i. Half-handstand at the Wall (*Ardha Adho Mukha Vrksasana*)

"Let's stand on our hands. Sit against the wall and note where your feet are. Put your palms at the spot and go into a small Down Dog with your feet against the wall. Walk your left foot and then your right foot up the wall. Make sure your hands are lined up under your shoulders. Can you walk your feet down the wall so you look like part of a square?"

Variation: Some people may feel comfortable doing a handstand against the wall with a partner to spot them. Find Down Dog, with your hands about eight inches from the wall. Walk your feet toward the wall, and then lift one leg and then the other. A person can spot someone by placing their hands on the person's hips as they kick up. Just make sure the spotter does not get kicked.

Challenge: Scorpion *(Vrischika)*

Reverse Half Handstand

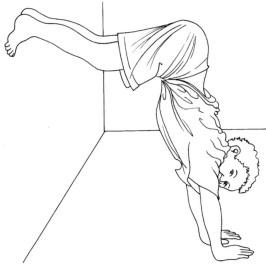

Reverse Half Handstand

Caution: This pose should only be done in small supervised groups with people who have been doing yoga for a while. It is a fun pose, but it is not appropriate for a large group or for beginners as it could cause injury.
   Facing the wall, rest your forearms on the mat, elbows lined up with your shoulders. Walk your feet toward your hips and lift up toward the wall so that your feet rest on the wall. Lift your chin away from the floor and breathe!

Benefits: These poses build arm and back strength. Reversing our position can also bring the added benefit of looking at things a new way!

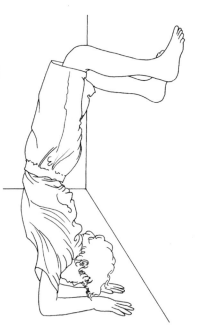

Scorpion

5. Twist and Shout: Spinal Twists

You are as young as your spine is healthy.
—Yoga saying

This section explores the six ways we can bend our spine and the reasons this keeps the body healthy. You can bend your spine forward (flexion); backward into a backbend (extension); twist to each side (rotation); and side bend to each side (lateral flexion). Moving the spine keeps the muscles and ligaments around the spine healthy and stimulates the spinal fluid. Gravity continually compresses the spine. Yoga can help create space between the bones in the spine, the vertebrae. By lengthening and aligning the spine, stress on other systems, for examples, musculoskeletal, digestive, respiratory, and circulatory are examples, is reduced.

Facts About You:

"We each have 26 vertebrae: seven in the neck (cervical); 12 in the chest area (thoracic), five at the base of the spine (lumbar); the sacrum (five fused vertebrae); and the coccyx, our vestigial tail, four fused vertebrae). Did you know you have the same number of vertebrae in your neck as a giraffe—seven! Let's see how many ways we can exercise our spines."

a. Cat *(Bidalasana)/***Cow** *(Bitilasana)/***Thread the Needle** *(Sucirandhrasana)*

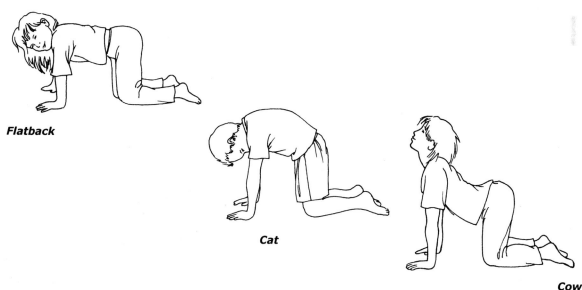

Flatback

Cat

Cow

"Let's warm up the spine and count how many ways we can move it. Find Flatback. Then take a deep breath in, then exhale and make a hissing sound as you arch your back up like a fierce cat. Then breathe in and moo as you let the belly sink toward the floor, like a swayback, sad and sorry cow. Do this three times. We just moved the spine two ways (flexion and extension). Come back to Flatback

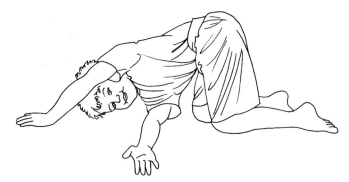

Now reach your right arm out, and as you take a breath out, thread it under your left arm. Your shoulder might touch the mat. Feel the stretch in your upper back. Hold this for two breaths, come back to Flatback, and do the other side. How did we just move the spine in that pose?"

Thread the Needle

Challenge: With the right shoulder toward the mat, extend the left leg toward the back of the room. Keep the foot flexed, as if you are kicking it into the wall.

Benefits: The pose helps keep the spine flexible and increases blood flow to the muscles that support the spine.

b. Forward Fold Twist

"Find Mountain Pose, take a deep breath in and sweep your arms to the sky. As you breathe out, bend your knees and bend forward so that your fingers or hands touch the floor. Now take a deep breath in and sweep your left hand to the sky. Feel the gentle twist as you lift that arm. Stay here for two breaths and then switch sides.

Variation: Reach your left hand to the sky and look toward it.

Challenge: As the right hand rests on the floor, reach the left arm around and grasp the top of your right hip, waistband, or thigh to deepen the twist.

Forward Fold Twist

Benefits: This forward fold brings length to the spine, using the weight of the head to create space between each vertebra. The lengthening of the spine gives the spinal nerves that exit more room so they do not get pinched. The slight twisting action helps keep the spine flexible.

c. Chair Pose Twist

"From mountain pose, imagine what it would feel like to sit down in a chair behind you—and then do it as you breathe out. Bring your hands into *Angeli mudra*, or palms to heart center. On your next breath out, turn and bring your right arm to the outside of your left knee. Take two breaths here, then you can melt down into a forward fold. Take a big breath in and lift your whole body toward the sky. Now let the other side of your body enjoy the same wonderful twist."

Challenge: Once in the pose, open the right arm up to the sky and the left arm to the floor. Do both sides. From Chair Prayer, unwind and stretch forward into Warrior 3. Then step back into a lunge. Step forward into chair and do the other side.

Benefits: The twist increases spinal flexibility and provides some cleansing for the abdominal organs as they are squeezed like a sponge. The kidneys, liver, stomach, and intestines are all compressed, and as the twist unwraps, they are infused with new blood.

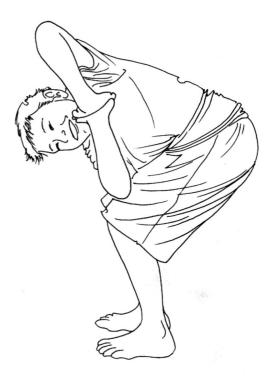

Chair Prayer

d. Twisted Prayer Lunge

"Let's see if we can twist the spine yet another way, to stretch out the tiny muscles between the vertebrae. From Mountain Pose, step the left foot back. You can be balancing on your toes or you can drop your left knee to the mat. Put your hands in *Angeli mudra*, or palms to heart center. Find your balance by pressing your palms together and lifting your chest off your leg as you turn open. Take a deep breath in and then twist to the right, resting the outside of your left arm on your right thigh. Take three breaths here, unwrap, and then lift back to Mountain Pose and do the other side."

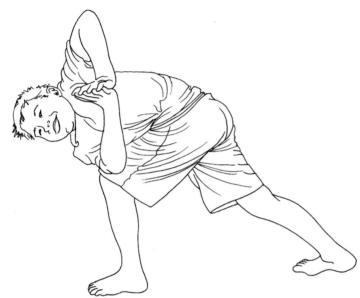

Twisted Prayer Lunge

Challenge: From this pose, open your arms out so that the right arm stretches to the sky and your left arm reaches toward the floor.

Benefits: The pose provides a wonderful stretch for the spine and an opportunity to practice balance. It stretches out the upper back and the core muscles. Twists also wring toxins out of the abdominal organs.

e. Spinal Twist 'n Kick

"Here is a pose that let's you balance, twist, and kick at the same time. Come to your hands and knees in Flatback. Extend your right arm out as if you were trying to reach something but you cannot quite reach. Extend your left leg back, as if you are kicking away the wall. Take a deep breath in, and as you breathe out, reach back and grab your left ankle and kick up into your right hand. Hold this for two breaths, release out but not down, then release back into Flatback. Now balance, kick and twist on the other side."

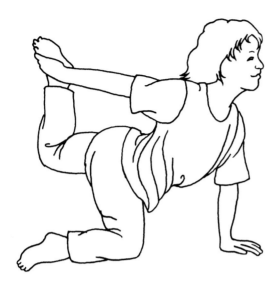

Spinal Twist'n Kick

Variation: Let's make the fierce cat and the sad cow move around—maybe the cat is chasing the cow! From Flatback, lift the right arm and left leg. Take a deep breath in, and on an exhale, tuck the right arm into the chest and bend your left knee in to meet your nose, which is tucking toward your chest.

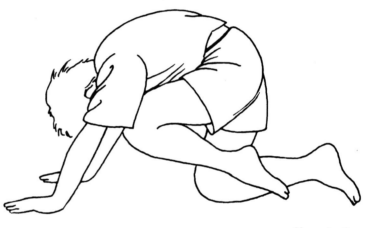

Nose to Knee

Breathe in and extend everything out again, then exhale and tuck. Do this four times on each side. In what way is the spine moving now? For another variation, lift the arm and the leg as high as you can before you exhale and tuck them close to your body.

Challenge: Find Flatback. Then raise your right hand and your right leg. After you find your balance, reach back and grab your right ankle with your right hand. Lift the leg and balance.

Benefits: This pose stretches out deep hip flexor muscles (psoas) on the lifted leg side, opens the chest, and flexes the spine.

f. Pretzel Parts

"Do you like your pretzels to be thin, thick, straight, bent, or salty? Let's try to twist like a twisted pretzel and see where your body allows you to go. Take a seat with your knees bent. Take a deep breath as you lift your spine toward the sky. As you breathe out, keep that lift in your spine and turn and look over your left shoulder as you bring your right elbow (or hand) to the outside of your left leg. Again, as you breathe in, lift the heart. As you breathe out, deepen your twist. Take three breaths here and then switch sides. Did you feel like a twisting pretzel?"

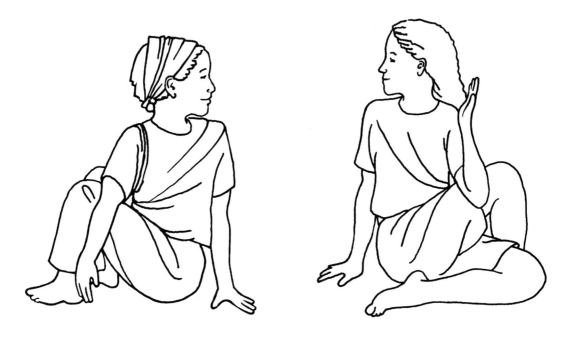

Pretzel Parts

Challenge: Move into a deeper twist by crossing your left leg over your right. Now extend your right hand around the outside of the left thigh and through the space under your left knee and reaching your left arm around back to grasp the right hand. Now that is a pretzel! Now do the other side.

Benefits: Twists are calming to the nervous system. This twist stretches the muscles on the outer hips. Doing both sides ensures that the body gets an even stretch, which helps to protect the joints.

g. Lying Down Twist

"Lying on your back, draw the right leg in and rest the sole of the right foot on the left thigh. Put the left hand on the outside of the right knee and take a deep breath in. As you breathe out, let the right knee melt over to the left, while you look out over your right hand. Stay here for four breaths—each time you breathe out try to melt a little deeper into the twist. Then do the other side."

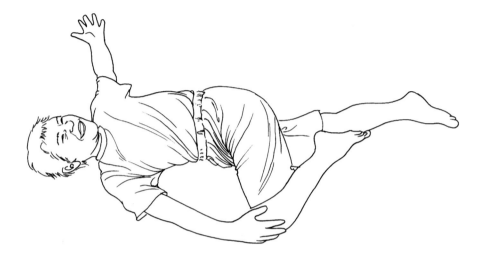

Lying Down Twist

Challenge: Lying on your back, bend both knees toward the chest. Cross the right knee over the left and catch the right foot behind the left calf. As you breathe out, allow the knees to melt over to the left, while you look over toward your right palm. Breathe here for four breaths, then change sides.

Benefits: Lying down twists stimulate the parasympathetic nervous system (the opposite of the sympathetic or the fight or flight response), which allows us to relax. The spine is lengthened as are the muscles in the core and along the outer leg.

6. Make the Connection

Yoga means yoking or union. The union can be as simple as touching your hands to your legs or as mysterious and wonderful as finding that our mind is indeed connected to our body. In yoga, it is the breath that can deepen the connection between the mind and the body.

Connections are all around us, from the connection of parts of our body, to connecting with one's friends and family, to the land that feeds us, to the water that sustains us, and to the air we breathe. So it is both easy and natural for people to enjoy yoga poses that celebrate their connection to all manner of things.

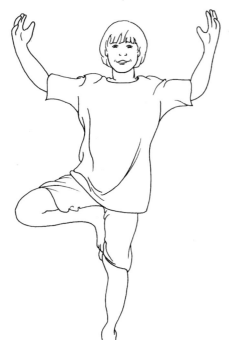

a. Tree Pose (*Vrksasana*): **Connect with the Earth**

"Connect with the earth by rooting yourself firmly into the ground on one foot. Imagine your favorite tree as you press the sole of your left foot into your right leg. Then be a different tree as you shift to the other foot. Can you connect with your friends and the earth by creating a forest as you link arms in a line or circle and all do tree pose together?
How is a tree connected the ground? To the air? To the water? To you?"

Challenge: Put your palms to heart center. Inhale the arms to the sky, and as you breathe out, extend the arms out to your side before bringing them back to your heart. Take up as much space as you can with this flowing movement as you use your breath in to lift the arms to the sky.

Tree Pose

Tree Pose

Benefits: Standing on one leg creates a feeling of rooting down into the earth for support and balance.

b. Forward Fold: Connect with Yourself

"From Mountain Pose, take a deep breath in through your nose and lift your arms to the sky. As you breathe out, bend forward to where your body wants to stop, and rest your hands on the tops of your shins. Take four breaths in this pose, lifting about one inch as you breathe in and melting down a little bit more each time you breathe out."

Challenge: As you bend forward, tuck your palms underneath your feet. Your knees can be bent, but as you inhale, allow them to straighten as you can.

Benefits: Forward folds stretch out the backs of the legs and the spine. A standing forward fold uses the weight of the head to deepen the spinal stretch.

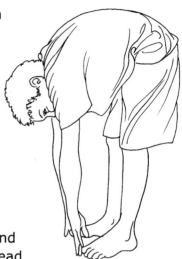

Forward Fold

c. Chair Pose *(Utkatasana)*: Connect with Your Breath

"Your breath is an important part of you, and you can connect with it by knowing where it is. It is easy—just pay attention to it as you move. Find Mountain Pose. Take a breath in and reach your hands to the sky. As you breathe out, take a seat. Keep the breath going and you will enjoy your new chair. It is so important not to hold your breath in a pose because that tells the body you feel stressed. Let's count how many breaths you can take as you sit in your new seat.

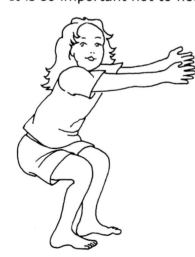

Variation: Keep the arms out in front of you, as if you are holding on to an exercise bar. Visualize holding onto that bar as you melt down into your chair. Once you are in Chair Pose, lift up onto your toes and sit down a bit more deeply.

Chair Pose

Chair Pose

Challenge: Use your breath in to lift your body back to Mountain Pose (or to just standing on one leg), and as you breathe out, extend forward into Warrior 3. On the next inhale, come back up on the standing leg and wrap the other leg around for Eagle Pose. (page 108) Use even breathing to keep the mind calm. For even more of a challenge, unwind and step back into a lunge.

Benefits: Focusing on the breath is a major tool in stress management. Counting the breaths in this pose keeps the attention on the breath and allows the person to use the breath to keep the mind calm.

d. Double Boat: *(Navasana)* Connect with A Friend

"Find a friend whose legs are about the same length as yours. Take each other's wrists, keeping your bent knees on the inside of your arms. Look at each other and take a breath in at the same time. Now put the soles of your feet together on one side and lift the legs. Now do the other side. Look at each other as you breathe in together and then breathe out together. Can you *feel* how you have connected to your breath and to the breath of your friend?"

Variation: Once everyone has found their Double Boats, can everyone breathe in together and then breathe out at the same time?

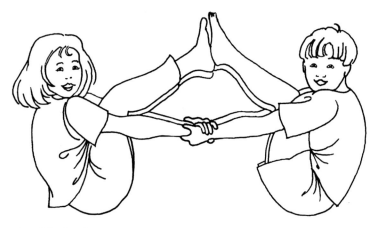

Double Boat

Challenge: Can you do the boat pose with four or five people?

Benefits: Physical contact with someone can be soothing by itself, and looking at them as they breathe reinforces the awareness of the breath. This is the first step to learning to keep the breathing even, a key to finding calm. This pose also brings a lot of laughter to the practice. Yael once had a duo of 7 year olds who stayed in the pose for 15 minutes, giggling and chatting quietly the whole time. The next class, they did it again—a practice for Yael in being open to kids' yoga!

e. Flower Pose: Connect with Friends

"Make one big circle and then sit down so that your knees are touching as you draw the soles of your feet together and lift your feet. Balance on your bottom for two breaths and then release the feet down. Weave your arms under your knees and grab the hand of the person on either side. Lift back up for a group balance."

Note: Some heavier people might not be able to weave their arms under their knees—just say, "The pose may work better for you if your arms stay above your knees, and feel free to rest your feet on the floor." The key, as always, is creating a safe environment for people to explore the possibilities.

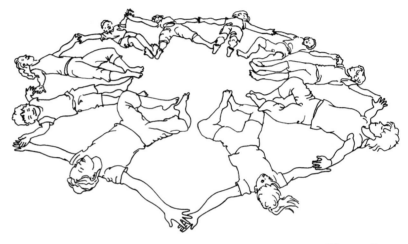

Flower Pose

Variation: Unwrap your arms and lift them overhead. Take a breath in and as you breathe out, let your body melt down to the floor. Reach out your arms and feet so they touch the hands and feet of the person on either side. Your group has just blossomed into a big flower. The largest flower in the world is the rafflesia, found in Southeast Asia—it can be three feet in diameter and weigh 24 pounds. It also smells like rotting meat to attract insects!

Take a breath and come back up into the balancing flower pose with the soles of your feet together, hands on your ankles. Then let your legs release and bend forward, just like a flower closing its petals. Imagine the sun warming you as you slowly breathe in and open out into a full flower bloom again.

Note: It is fun to add the SOLA Circle to this section, (see p. 162)

Benefits: As social creatures, we appreciate being part of a happy group. This pose creates a positive environment for everyone. If the rest of the day is stressful, perhaps the happy Flower Pose is something a person can remember as a bright spot of the day. This pose is the most requested pose in most classes.

7. Take Up Space

People who study space, the area around us, use a lot of interesting words, like quark and lepton, and wonder if space if curved or flat. In yoga, we try to stretch our bodies and lengthen our muscles so we take up more space, even while scientists are still trying to figure out what space really is! Let's use our breath to help us create even more space within our body. As you breathe in, lengthen your muscles and bones. As you breathe out, try to keep that length you have created. As we breathe in again, imagine the breath creating more space between your joints, the spaces between the bones.

a. Tall Mountain *(Tadasana)*

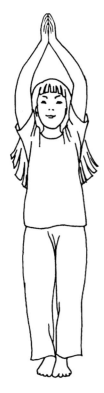

"Stand in Mountain Pose. What is the tallest point in our state? How could you be taller? Breathe in and lift your arms as high as you can. How could you be even taller? Keep stretching up as you lift up onto your toes and lengthen your whole body toward the sky. Create as much space in your body as you can by taking in another deep breath."

Challenge: As you breathe in and lift up on your toes, close your eyes.

Benefits: Visualizing using the breath to create space in the body helps develop the connection between the breath and the body. Stretching up lengthens the muscles in the legs, the core, the back, and the arms.

b. Star Pose

"From Mountain Pose, step your feet apart and lift your arms overhead so that you look like a giant letter X. Take up as much space as you can by spreading your fingers wide and pressing out at the same time you press your feet into the earth. Think about a star radiating heat and light. Lift your heart a little higher as you press down with your feet."

Tall Mountain

Variation: Try this pose lying down.

Challenge: Take up even more space by standing on your tip toes.

Benefits: This pose strengthens the legs and opens the chest to receive a full breath.

c. Warrior 2 to Reverse Warrior 2

"From Mountain Pose, step your left foot back and spin it flat. Take a bend in the front knee and then lift your arms like a "T". Think about lifting up from under your ribs, so you can find even more length in your Warrior." Then turn the right paum up and bend back to reverse warrior.

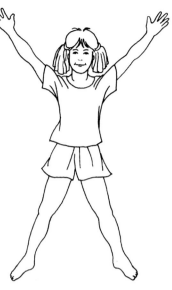

Star Pose

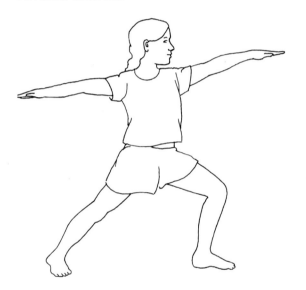

Warrior 2

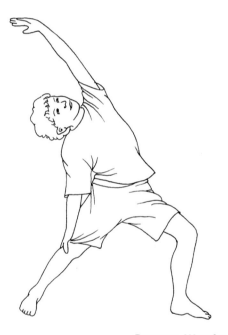

Reverse Warrior 2

Challenge: After Reverse Warrior 2, shift your weight forward over your front leg and come forward into Half Moon. With your right hand on the floor, keep your left hand on your left hip and you stack your hips, one above the other. When you feel as if your bones are stacked tall, then breathe in and lift your left arm to the sky (this does not need to be done at the wall).

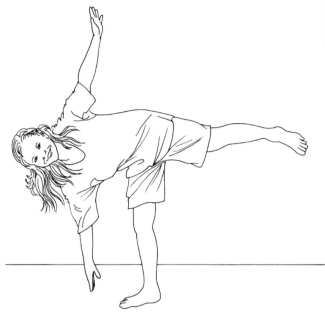

Benefits: This pose strengthens the legs, lengthens the spine, and opens the chest.

Half Moon

d. Wide-legged Down Dog *(Prasarita Adho mukha svanasana)*

"How could we make Down Dog take up even more space? How about if we widen the space between our feet? Find a Down Dog pose and move your feet apart. Lift your hips toward the sky and bark three times like a dog you know."

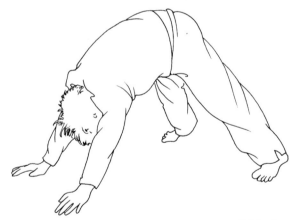

Wide-legged Down Dog

Benefits: Doing a familiar pose with a slight variation often draws our attention back to how the pose is making us feel. The wide-legged stance builds strength and stimulates the flow of lymph, the fluid of our immune system.

e. Wide-legged Up Dog *(Prasarita Urdhva mukha svanasana)*

"From wide-legged Down Dog, move forward so that your shoulders are over your wrists in a plank. Press back through your heels and keep your hips from melting toward the ground. The take a deep breath in as you curl up into Wide-Legged Up Dog."

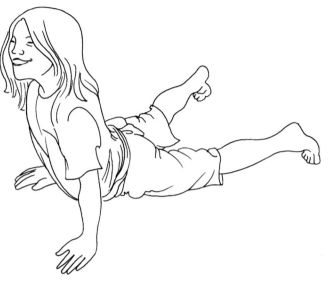

Wide-legged Up Dog

Challenge: Take up even more space by making your body flow from wide-legged Down Dog to wide-legged Plank to wide-legged Up Dog (let your hips melt toward the floor). On a breath out, lift back into wide-legged down dog and do the flow two more times. Feel your body build the heat (tapas)—that is a good thing as it allows your muscles to lengthen and cleanses the body of toxins.

Benefits: Wide-legged Plank and Up Dog build shoulder and core strength.

C. More Yoga Games

By definition, games provide entertainment or amusement. Yoga lends itself to games because yoga can be both entertaining and amusing. And since everyone loves to play games, we invite you to mix these yoga games into any practice to add more flavor and fun.

1. Wobble Alert: Green, Yellow, and Red Alert!

Doing some balance poses at the beginning of a practice is a great way to get everyone's attention. It helps clear the mind as people try to focus on keeping their balance. Use these three poses as your "Wobble Alert Game" after you have set your intentions for the practice.

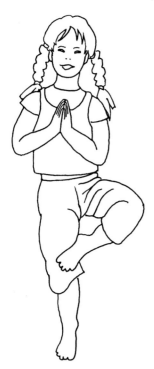

a. Tree Pose *(Vrksasana)*: **Green Alert**

"Is there any wind in here? So our trees should not be wobbling in the wind. Shift your weight to your right foot and lift the left leg so that you can press the sole of the left foot into your right calf or thigh (not the knee). If you wobble, rest your big toe on the ground. Find your wobble-free zone and then try again on the other side."

b. Bush Pose: Yellow Alert

"Let's try more of a challenge, the Yellow Alert Bush Pose. Shift your weight to your right foot and cross your left foot over your right knee. Keep your left foot flexed, as if you are standing on the ground. Put your palms to heart center, take a deep breath in, and as you can, melt down so you become a smaller bush. Hold for two breaths, unwind, and do the other side."

Tree Pose

Tree Pose

c. Warrior Three: Red Alert!

"Let's see if you wobble on this Red Alert pose, a very challenging balance pose. From Mountain Pose, shift your weight on to your right foot. Inhale your arms to the sky, and as you breathe out, extend forward so your body looks like the letter T. If you want to rest your back toes on the mat for your Warrior 3, that is fine. Remember, yoga is about finding your stretch, not someone else's."

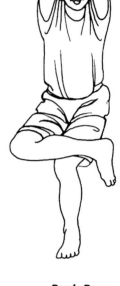

Bush Pose

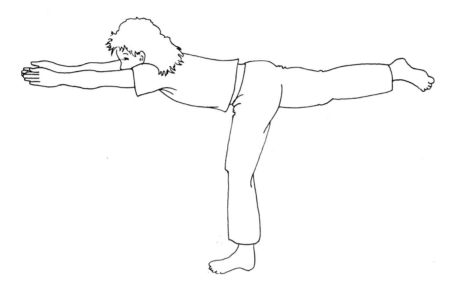

Warrior 3

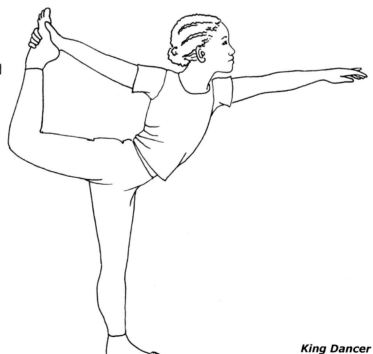

Challenge: From Warrior 3, reach back with your left hand and grasp the left ankle for King Dancer Pose.

Benefits: The series builds focus and concentration. In addition, the standing balance poses strengthen muscles in the standing leg, the core, and the gluteal muscles.

King Dancer

2. To Focus or not to Focus . . .

"A wonderful benefit of yoga is the practice of developing focus or concentration. This simple and fun exercise allows people to use their own bodies to demonstrate the power of their minds. Go through each of the "Wobble Alert" Poses, but with the following variation. Before you start each pose, make sure everyone finds a *drishti* point, a focus point at eye level. They will "fix their gaze" on that point and not break their gaze as everyone does Tree Pose. Then have one person stand, without moving his feet, at the front of someone else's mat. Instruct that person to make all sorts of funny faces and wave their hands—but without making any noises. Now try to do that same Tree Pose again, amid all the distraction. Have them note the difference. What changed? Switch partners.

Benefits: In addition to the benefits of standing balance poses, this series helps develop social skills as people work in partners. It also allows people the opportunity to laugh—a great way to relieve stress by lowering cortisol (a stress hormone) levels in the blood.

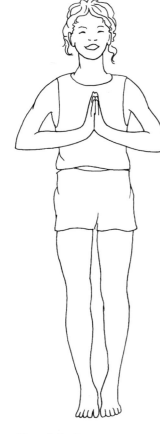

3. Get Pumping

"Get Pumping" draws awareness to the heart by counting heartbeats in a resting pose and followed by more energizing poses.

a. Mountain Pose *(Tadasana)*

"Stand in Mountain Pose and put your hand over your heart. Can you feel it beat? Now count the number of beats in 20 seconds. Remember that number. When you exercise, your body needs to bring more oxygen to your muscle cells so they can move. So your heart beats faster to pump the blood all around your body. Do you still remember the number of heartbeats in 20 seconds or should we count again? We are going to move through a sun salutation, or a salute to the sun, which is the energy source for our whole planet. What do you think will happen to your heart beats?"

Mountain Pose

b. Forward Fold *(Uttanasana)*

"Take a deep breath in and as you breathe out, bend forward and touch your shins or the mat."

c. Flat Back *(Ardha Uttanasana)*

"Breath in and lift your heart so your back is flat, let the breath out and fold forward again."

d. Lunge

"Step your right foot back and find a straight-legged lunge with your hands on either side of your front foot. The back leg can be up or the knee can rest on the mat"

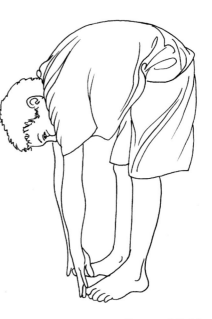

Forward Fold

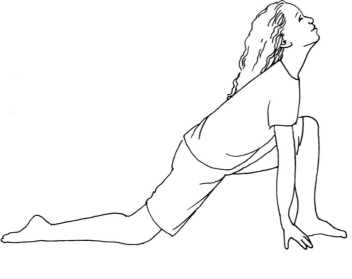

Lunge

e. Down Dog *(Adho mukha svanasana)*

"Step the other foot back and lift your hips to find your Down Dog."

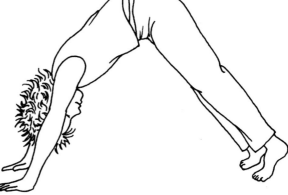

Down Dog

89

f. Plank

Breathe in and come forward into a plank position, pressing back through your heels and keeping your back straight like a plank or a board.

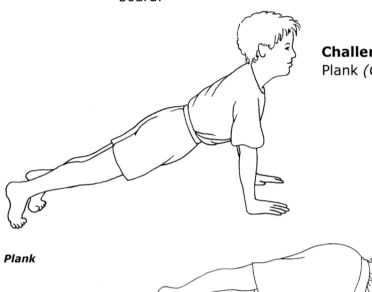

Challenge: Lower down into Low Plank (*Chataranga Dandasana*)

Plank

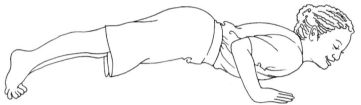

Low Plank

g. Cobra (*Bhujangasana*)

"Drop your knees and lift your heart into a high cobra pose. Curl the toes under and push back into Down Dog."

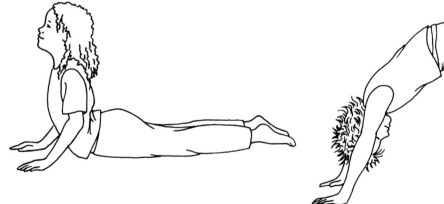

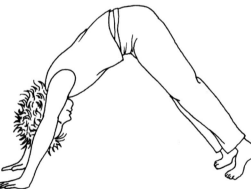

Cobra

Down Dog

h. Warrior 1 *(Virabhadrasana)*

"Step your right foot forward into a lunge and then take a breath in and reach you arms toward the sky. Exhale your hand back down to the mat. Like a wave coming into shore, sweep your left foot up between your hands and stand in forward fold."

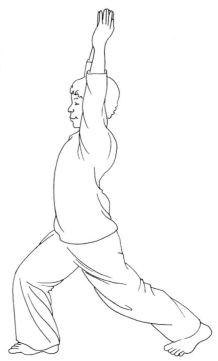

Warrior 1

i. Mountain Pose *(Tadasana)*

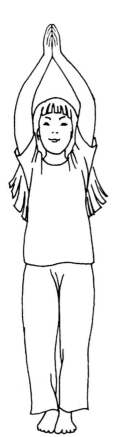

"Sweep your hands up into tall Mountain Pose, then put your palms to heart center.

Now count the number of times your heart beats in 20 seconds. Did your heart rate go up or go down? Why do you know it changed? Let's do the sun salutation on the other side (stepping the left foot back in the first lunge) and see what happens."

Tall Mountain

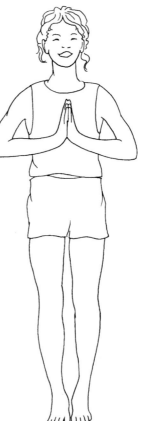

Mountain Prayer

4. Keep on Counting

Keep On Counting helps bring the awareness to the breath by using calming poses juxtaposed to highly energetic ones.

"Let's keep counting your heartbeats. Remember the number of times your heart beat after the sun salutations we just did. (Or you can count the heartbeats after any group of poses that are quite active.) Now we are going to do three poses and then see what has changed with our hearts."

a. Child's Pose (*Balasana*) **or Extended Child's Pose**

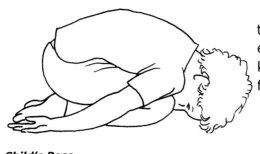

"Sit back on your heels with your big toes touching and your knees out toward the edge of your mat. Let your chest rest on your knees as you close your eyes and settle down for five rounds of breath."

Child's Pose

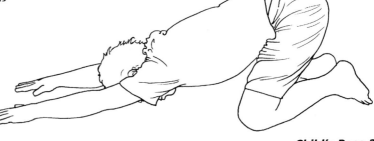

Child's Pose 2

b. Back To Breathing

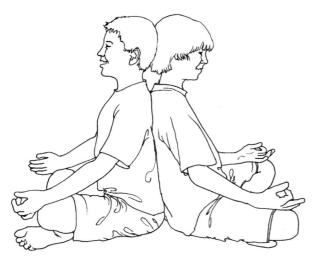

"Sit in Easy Pose with your back to a partner's back. Close your eyes and breathe in together, so you can feel the other person's back press into your back as she breathes in. Then breathe out through your mouth, so you can hear it, together."

Back to Breathing

c. Butterfly *(Baddha Konasana)*

"Now sit with the soles of your feet together. Grasp your ankles, close your eyes, and take a deep breath in as you lift your chest. Take three breaths here.

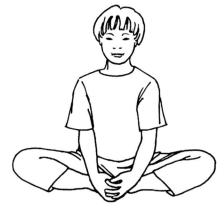

Butterfly

Now count your heartbeats. Did the number of beats go up or down? Why do you think it changed?"

5. Flex time: Butterfly Press

Flex Time plays with the PNF response (Proprioceptive Neuromuscular Facilitation) in a way that makes everyone laugh as they can watch it happening in their own bodies! PNF is part of flexibility training, using the contracting and then relaxing of a muscle to allow for a deeper stretch. Lilias Folan uses it as a tool to teach and writes about it, calling it part of the 3 Rs—"Resist, Relax, and Restretch." As Lilias says, "The three Rs are a creative way to listen to your body. Listening to your body is a life-long journey."[19] Games are a fun way for people to develop awareness of their own bodies.

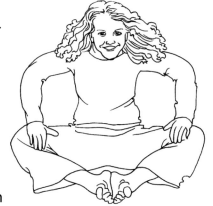

"Sit with the soles of your feet together. Gently drop your knees toward the floor. Just notice where the knees stop. They probably will not touch the floor, and that is fine. Let's play with the muscles. Gently press your palms against your knees at the same time you push your knees back up. Take four breaths pressing the palms down as the knees press up. The knees won't move! Then release the hands, and watch what happens."

Butterfly Press

93

6. Yoga Word Searches

Check our website (Greentreeyoga) for Yoga Word Searches and Yoga Crossword Puzzles for Grades 1-3 and Grades 4-6. Print them out and have some fun.

7. New Pose Contest

A fifth grader developed this pose and named it Wolf Pose. It is a wonderful way to stretch the quadriceps, the tops of the feet and the toes, and open the chest. It also opens the throat and stimulates the lymph as you howl, just as when you roar in Lion Pose! See what your body comes up with and let us know. You could win a free book or a yoga mat. Your pose will get shown on our website too. Go to our website and send us an email with your ideas.

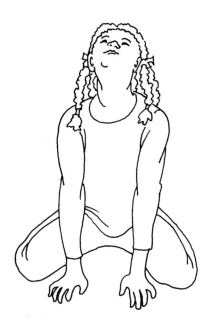

Wolf Pose

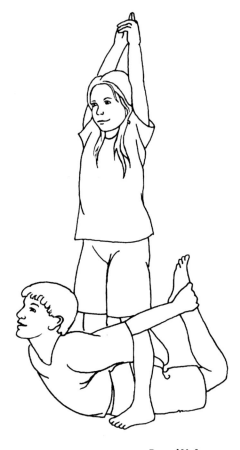

For another contest to win prizes, Designing a SOLA Yoga Stikk, **See page 146**

Bow 'N Arrow

D. Relaxation

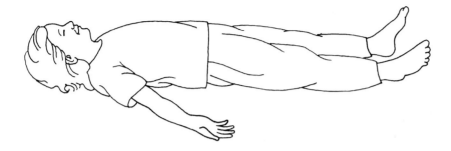

Savasana: Final Relaxaton

Final Relaxation is a key part of any yoga practice. For some young people, it may even be their favorite part. Yael has had many students say, "When do we get to the lying down part?" Everyone likes permission to just "be"—to just allow their minds and their bodies to be free from demands, requests, or suggestions for a bit.

Relaxation, or bringing ease to the mind, is the intention of any yoga practice. Yoga poses—Warrior, Crow, Mountain, and Down dog—help to stretch and strengthen muscles so that the body can then be still, without wiggles or fidgeting, for a while. When the body is at ease, we can find ease in the mind. We use the breath to help get us to that point of relaxation or ease of mind in a reliable way. So we end a yoga practice with the celebration of that relaxation state—with the pause in active movement and thought. We invite you to take the opportunity to show young people how that can feel.

In doing active poses, the relaxing muscles can feel warm or tingle. But as we lie still in final relaxation, it may be appropriate for people to put on their socks or a second shirt if they have it. When the body stops moving, it cools down. It is nice to keep a warm feeling in final relaxation.

So please leave time at the end of every practice, at least five to ten minutes, for Final Relaxation. The following is a simple relaxation, bound to please and quick to become a favorite. There are more relaxation exercises in Section III.

The following is from the book *Create a Yoga Practice for Kids* (Sunstone Press, 2006). It is offered again because it is so popular. It has been known to put kids to sleep in five minutes— and if done over time the kids will burst into the yoga class and offer a new rhyme. And, Yael has had parents ask her for this poem (written by Uncle Matthew and evolved, like folk art, over many years as a bedtime poem for Yael's three active boys!) to hang on their kids' wall. This rhyming poem is easy to memorize. Just start at the feet and work your way up to the head. Have fun with it.

"Listen as I help you to relax the rest of you."
(Say this slowly, finding a lilting, soothing, unrushed rhythm so people have time to relax with each part.)

"Wiggle your toes, then let them doze,
Relax your feet to this gentle beat,
Relax your heels, like sunning seals
Relax your legs like mama birds sitting on eggs
Relax your knees, just say please
Relax your hips, don't do flips
Relax your bones, with gentle tones
Relax your muscles, from their tussles
Relax your nerves, with healing herbs
Relax your tummy, just say yummy
Relax your heart, it's a good start
Relax your ribs, like babies' bibs
Relax your chest, let it rest
Relax your back, like a cuddle sack
Relax your back, your neck and spine
Relax your spine like a tall limber pine
Relax your trapezius 'cuz it's the easiest
Relax each shoulder before you get older
Relax your arms with wizards' charms
Relax each elbow, let them swing low
Relax each hand without a demand
Relax each finger, yet them linger
Relax each palm, like a gentle psalm
Relax your jaw, let it thaw
Relax your nose, let it doze
Relax your skin, tuck it in
Relax your chin, just as your skin
Relax your mind, in front and behind
Relax your face, like silk and lace
Relax your eyes, like warm summer skies
Relax your ears with joyful tears
Relax your brain like a gentle spring rain"
(The last line for bedtime is "And put your head, gently to bed.)

After a few minutes say, "Now slowly start to wiggle your fingers and toes. Stretch your hands over your head and stretch from tip to toe. Still with your eyes closed, bring your knees into your chest and roll over on to your side. Count four breaths. Remember a breath is a full inhale and a full exhale. When you are ready, still with your eyes closed, help yourself up to sitting and sit in Easy Pose.

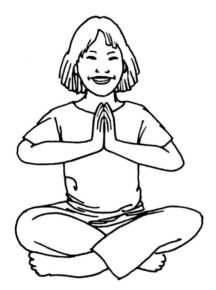

Easy Pose

The last part of a yoga practice is to place your hands together in *Angali mudra* and bow to each other. Together we say, *Namaste*, which means, 'The goodness in me bows to, or acknowledges, the goodness in you.' We all have goodness in us, and it is nice when someone else notices it!

When you need to help yourself calm down, listening for your breath is a way to let a feeling of relaxation come to you."

Benefits: Final Relaxation allows kids to just let go—they learn that they can create a calmness within themselves. Doing Final Relaxation with some guided activity in the beginning invites kids to become a part of the process and practice the powerful tool of visualization.

E. Five Minute Yoga in Any Classroom *

The right word may be effective, but no word was ever as effective as a rightly timed pause.
—Mark Twain

Yoga can be used to create a short break in a classroom of students from elementary to high school—although Yael also uses yoga breaks in her college lecture (not yoga) classes. We were asked by schools to develop "Five Minute Yoga" breaks to offer teachers a way to meet some state's physical education requirements and to help improve the classroom learning environment. Having students become familiar with a short flow helps ease those challenging transition points of any school day. By repeating the breaks each day, they become both an energizing and calming routine.

Yael worked many years as a classroom teacher and knows the dynamics of a school day. She also uses two minute yoga breaks when doing programs on other topics in her children's schools. For example, when doing a holiday program for 100 first graders or presenting science fair topics to fifth graders (both one hour programs), she would break up the program with two minutes of standing yoga every time kids got fidgety.

* Available on CD by Green Tree Yoga.

Yoga as a Classroom Management Tool:

A yoga break gives the students a tool to take with them to use at home or in other classes. Yael had a fourth grader in an after school yoga class who came running in one day, saying, "What was that yoga pose you said we could do when we were feeling stressed in class?" She had not remembered the pose, just that yoga was a tool to help her. And keep in mind that these yoga breaks will make you, the teacher, feel better too.

Use these yoga breaks as a tool for both you and your students to:

◇ Calm down
◇ Perk up
◇ Focus and concentrate
◇ Relieve stress
◇ Be more positive about learning
◇ Smile!

Remember the Breath.

Using the breath, while at rest and while moving, is a key to accessing the benefits of yoga. So as you lead your class in these series of fun poses, remember to prompt them to, "Breathe in as you lift your arms to the sky," or to "Push out all the breath as you bend forward." This attention to breathing out deeply allows people to take in much more fresh air, making them more alert and more relaxed. Remember that a breath has two parts—a full inhale and a full exhale. Also mention that yoga breathing is done through the nose, as it warms, lengthens, and cleans the breath. You can even have the students give an occasional audible sigh, as in "ahhh" when they exhale—a favorite release technique of Lilias Folan's to deepen relaxation. Read more about the importance of breath to help one relax and to focus on **pages 27–28.**

Remember the Pause:

*The notes I handle no better than many pianists. But the pauses between the notes—ah, that is where the art resides!
—Arthur Schnabel*

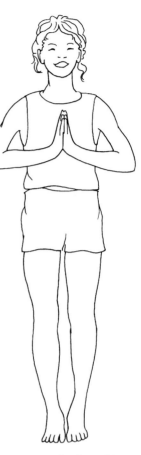

Reduce Stress and Be More Positive

These are designed to be five minutes breaks in your day. Because you are giving a gift to both yourself and your students, do not rush through your words. Just as in teaching your subjects, remember to pause and give students time to absorb what you have said, time for the body to respond by stretching and calming.

Be Flexible:

If you do not feel comfortable at first, perhaps there is a student or a yoga parent who would like to lead the five minute break. Often a good classroom management tool is to give a disruptive student a positive role in the class to get things back on the right track. Sometimes a parent or grandparent does yoga and would be happy to drop by your class (or several interested teachers' classes) to lead a five minute break. Take advantage of kids' natural affinity for yoga and make it part of your day.

Remember Visualization:

Please reread the paragraph on the power of visualization on **page 24.** It is wonderful to incorporate into a classroom, especially with students in whom you are trying to build self-confidence and a positive outlook on the possibilities for their own success.

Yoga Breaks:
Don't move the furniture, don't take off your shoes, just take a break!

We invite you to let yoga works its magic in your classroom. These poses are to stretch muscles and to get oxygen flowing after sitting for too long. They also bring laughter, always a stress release. But you can quickly regain quiet with the "Listen for Your Breath" trick for getting everyone quiet: palms to heart center, eyes closed, listening for your own breath. This calms both the mind and the body (and the teacher).

Consider these four distinct times that yoga can strengthen a busy classroom program.

1. To Open the Day:
A yoga break offers the class time to settle into the morning and to find a positive point from which to jump into the school day.

2. After Lunch:
A yoga break again provides a tool to bring students back to work through some calming, focusing physical movements. Yoga prepares the mind and the body for an afternoon of reading and learning.

3. To Close the Day:
Yoga provides the opportunity to end the day on a positive note, giving students the tool to find a bit of calm to take with them as they leave the school.

4. The Yoga Study Break
This yoga break can be used any time to turn the day around. If students are sleepy or restless or stressed or fidgety, this break can provide both the physical and mental break they need to get back on task with a positive approach. This break uses more standing poses, a good antidote to too much sitting.

1. To Open the Day

a. Seated breathing (in a chair or in a seated circle)

"Since we are going to be learning together today, let's start our day by breathing together. Slide forward in your chair so you can feel your back straighten. You can close your eyes if you like. Let's all take a deep breath in and as we breathe out, keep the lift in your spine. Breathe in again as we sweep our arms to the sky. Let's all breathe out as we let our arms very slowly float down. Let's do this three times to wake up the shoulders and the mind."

b. Set Intention for the Day (in a chair or in a seated circle)

"Intentions are a direction you would like to go, not a specific goal. So an intention could be to try your best in math today, to make your paper neater than yesterday, or to be nice to someone when you may not really feel like it. Put your hands together in front of your heart, close your eyes, and think to yourself what you would like your intention to be for today. Then take a deep breath in as you reach your hands toward the sky and open your eyes."

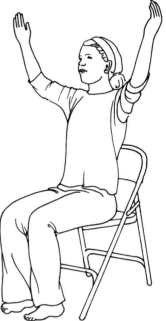

Seated Breathing

The Sanksrit word for intention is *sankalpa.* At some point, solicit ideas from the students as to possible intentions. You can also say later in the day, "Take a moment to check in with your intention for today." A gentle reminder might be just what someone needs to work more neatly or smile at someone.

c. Crescent Moon

"Before we begin stretching our minds, let's stretch out our bodies. Stand tall next to your chair. Take a breath in and grasp your right wrist with your left hand. Reach for the sky and then breathe out as you arc over to the left—feel your right foot pressing into the earth. What is something about you that shines today? (your smile, your colorful shirt, your happy attitude?) Like a bright moon, feel the light shining out of you." Do the other side. Repeat.

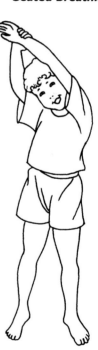

Crescent Moon.

101

d. Tree Pose *(Vrksanana)*

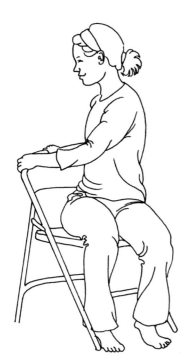

"Let's get our mind focused by waking up the cerebellum, the part of your brain that helps us to balance. Stand on your right foot, and press the sole of your left foot against your right calf or thigh (not knee). You can press your palms together, take a breath in as you reach for the sky. To really practice focus, close your eyes." Take two breaths and then switch sides.

e. Seated Half Moon

"Let's sit and find a bit more stretch. Put your left hand on your seat, and reach your right hand to the sky as you breathe in. Let your heart lift so all the light can shine out. Did you already shine your light on someone this morning? Who might you shine your light on later today?" Take two breaths here and then switch sides."

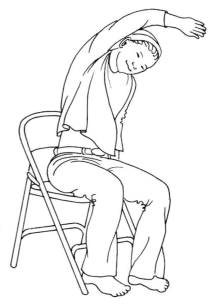

Tree Pose

Seated Half Moon

f. Seated Twist

"Reach back with your right hand and give your spine a pat. To take care of the spine and help keep it healthy, let's give it a gentle twist. Scoot forward in your seat and feel your spine lift as you do. Take a big breath in, and then as you breathe out, reach your right hand around to the left and grab the top of your chair. Stay here for two breaths, giving your spine time to move in a new way." Do the other side.

g. Listen for Your Breath

"Sit tall in your seat and bring your hands to heart center. Close your eyes and listen for your own breath. After four breaths (a breath is a full inhale and a full exhale), open your eyes. We have an intention, we stretched our bodies, we filled our lungs with oxygen, and now we are ready to begin our day!

Seated Twist

2. After Lunch

a. Mountain Pose *(Tadasana)*

"We have been moving around at lunch (and recess), so now let's be still and strong like the Rocky or Himalaya mountains. Actually, these mountains are slowly growing each day as they push up from the earth, so as you stand tall, see if you can use your breath and grow a bit. How could you be even taller (arms up, stand on tip toes)? Take three breaths in your strong mountain pose."

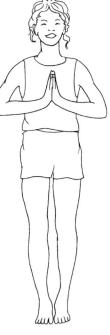

Mountain Pose

b. Standing Crescent Moon

"Before we return to stretching our minds, let's stretch and release some muscles in our body. Stand tall next to your chair. Take a breath in and reach your right hand to the sky and arc over to the left—press your right foot into the earth. Like a bright moon, feel the light shining out of you." Then do the other side. Repeat.

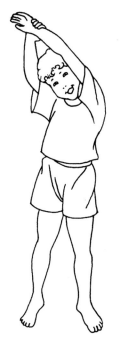

Crescent Moon.

c. Tree Pose *(Vrksasana)*

"Now let's exercise the mind by using the body. Does anyone have an idea about what that might mean? Stand on your right foot, and press the sole of your left foot against your right calf or thigh (not knee). You can press your palms together or reach for the sky. It takes extra concentration, a mind exercise, to do this pose with your eyes closed!" Take two breaths and then switch sides.

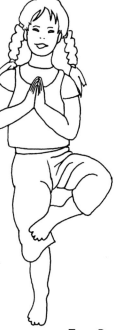

Tree Pose

d. Chair Pose (Utkasana)

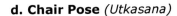

"Let's take a seat—but wait—without a chair. On your next breath in, lift your arms to the sky, breathe out and sit back. Stay here for two breaths, come up to Mountain Pose. Make yourself a chair one more time before you actually do sit in your chair."

You can also extend your arms out in front of you as if you are holding on to an exercise bar and then sit back.

Chair pose

e. Seated Forward Fold

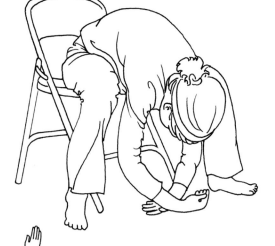

Seated Forward Fold

"Puff up your chest like a pigeon as you fill your lungs with air, and as you breathe out, sigh with an "aahh" and bend forward, putting our head in a new spot to get us thinking for the afternoon. Let your neck hang down gently. Take three breaths here and slowly take a deep breath in as you sit back up."

f. Seated Breathing

"Finally, let's use our breath to settle into our afternoon. Slide forward in your chair so you can feel your back straighten. Take a deep breath in and as you breathe out, keep the lift in your spine. On your next breath in, sweep your arms to the sky like a (let them fill in the analogy!). In slow motion, let your arms float down to your lap on the breath out. Do this two more times to settle the body and the mind into our afternoon activities."

Seated Breathing

3. To Close the Day

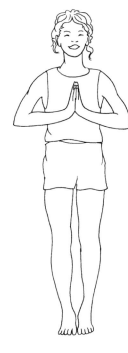

a. Mountain Pose
(Tadasana)

"Imagine a
mountain you
would like to visit.
What season is it?
Close your eyes
and stand tall like
that mountain. Take
three breaths in your
strong Mountain Pose."

Mountain Pose.

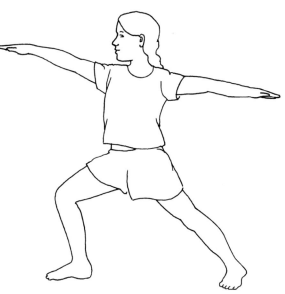

b. Warrior 2 *(Virabhadrasana 2)*

"Step your left foot back. Extend your arms out
like a T, while you look over your front middle finger.
As you breathe out, let the front knee bend, but keep
your body upright—do not let your chest lean forward.
Think about one thing you would like to be strong for
later today as you hold this pose for three breaths."
Do the other side and come back to Mountain Pose.

Warrior 2

c. Warrior 1 *(Virabhadrasana 1)*

"Now let's be another strong warrior by
stretching up because it helps keep the muscles
and the joints healthy. Step back and turn onto the
back toes as you swing your hips forward, like two
headlights shining in front of you. Lift your arms
to the sky and feel your own strength. Take three
breaths here and do the other side."

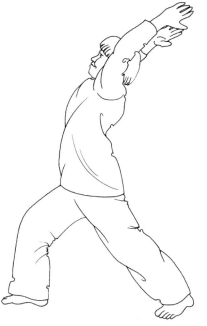

Warrior 1

d. Seated Breathing

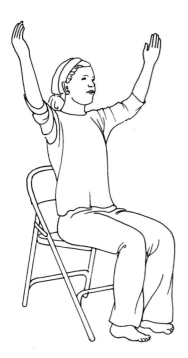

"Before you head home for the rest of your day, let's breathe together. Slide forward in your chair so you can feel your back straighten. You can close your eyes if you like and think of something good that happened today. Let's all take a deep breath in and as we breathe out, keep the lift in your spine. Breathe in again as we sweep our arms to the sky. Then breathe out as we let our arms slowly float down. Do this two more times. Notice how you feel, and remember that should you get upset later today, you can use your breath to calm you down. Just put your hand on you belly and feel your breath to help you relax."

e. Intention Check

"Rest your hands in your lap, close your eyes, and let yourself know if you met your intention for your day. (You can remind them of some options for intentions, perhaps planting a seed for setting an intention tomorrow.)

Seated Breathing

4. A Study Break

Inward calm cannot be maintained unless physical strength is constantly and intelligently replenished.
—Buddha

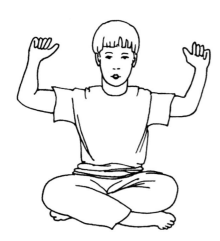

a. Bellows breathing (seated in chair)

"Sometimes you feel tired because your body is not getting enough oxygen—that is why you yawn. Let's take a yoga break by moving oxygen into our bodies. Find a comfortable spot on your chair. Lift your arms and fill your lungs with air. Now lower your arms in a quick motion while you push all the breath out of your body. Let's do this three times."

Bellows Breathing

b. Shoulder rolls (seated in chair)

"Move around in your chair a little to get a good, comfortable seat. You can bring some relaxation to your neck and shoulders. Pretend you have your favorite color marker on you elbow. Draw a circle with it by rolling the right shoulder forward three times, then roll it back. Now do the left shoulder. Now pick a color that makes you feel like jumping around. Imagine that on the end of your finger as you move your straight arm in circles, first three times forward and then three times backward to stretch out that shoulder. Now do the other side." Ask the students for ideas on what colors to choose—a color that makes them feel silly, sad, happy . . .

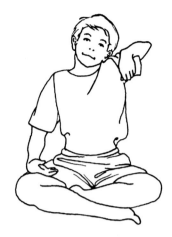

Shoulder Rolls

c. Chair Pose *(Utkasana)*

"Feel how strong your chair is. Now let's sit by using our strong muscles and not our chairs to hold us up. Stand up, and on your next breath in, lift your arms to the sky, breathe out and sit back. Stay here for two breaths, come up to Mountain Pose. Do one more chair before you do sit in your chair."

Note: You can also extend your arms in front of you as if you are holding on to an exercise bar and then sit back.

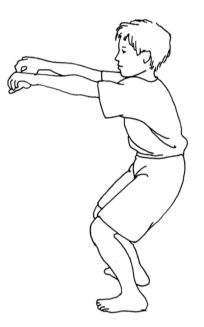

Chair Pose

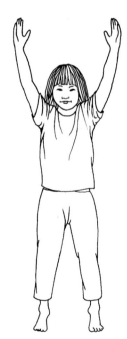

d. Rooster

"Let's get the blood flowing and muscles strengthening in the legs and feet. Stand in Mountain Pose. On a breath in, stand on your tip toes. Come down as you breathe out. Let your breath lift you up and down ten times."

Note: If you want to use more muscles, you can lift your arms as you come onto the tiptoes. If you want to use more of your brain, close your eyes.

Rooster

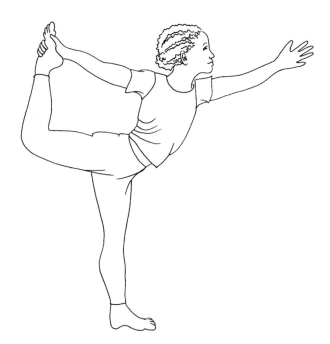

e. Standing Bow

"Let's stretch out the whole body now, and use the body to exercise the mind as we practice balance. Stand in Mountain Pose. Fix your gaze on a point at eye level that is not moving (a *drishti* point). Do not let your right foot move, while you lift your left leg and reach back to grasp your left ankle. Breathe out as you bend forward into a strong King Dancer. Stay here for three breaths and feel the muscles warming and the mind focusing on not falling! Come to mountain pose and listen for your breath. Then do the other side.

Standing Bow

f. Eagle *(Garudasana)*

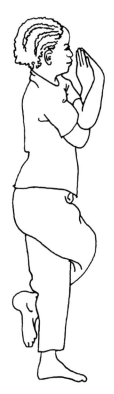

"The eagle is our national bird—why do you think that is? Find your Mountain Pose and a focus point at eye level. Stand on your right foot while you wrap your left foot around the right calf. If you like, put your palms together at your heart. Or you can extend your arms to the front and wrap your right arm over your left arm and clasp hands. Can you raise your hands in front of your face like a sharp eagle bill? Now, to really exercise your mind, practice your balance by sitting down a little bit. Take three breaths here. This pose strengthens and stretches so many important muscles. Now let's do the other side."

h. Number 4 Pose

"Instead of writing a number on paper, let's have our bodies *be* the number. This pose will stretch out the hip muscles, which

Eagle Pose

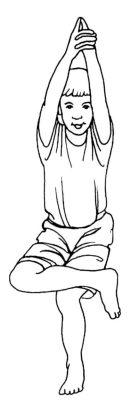

Number Four Pose

can get stiff when you sit too long. Stand in Mountain Pose. Cross your left foot over the top of your right knee. Keep the left foot flexed, as if it were still standing on the floor. Take a deep breath in and sit down into the pose. Take three more breaths and switch sides."

i. Hanging Bridge

Note: This is a partner pose, which can be done standing by a desk. It will generate a lot of laughter, which is a great way to turn the mood around or break up a stressful afternoon. It is very easy to get everyone quiet again by explaining that after the pose, we will all sit down and "Listen for Your Breath." Another way to keep more control is to have everyone get into the first part of the pose, then listen to you as you say, "Let's all take a breath in together, then breathe out together."

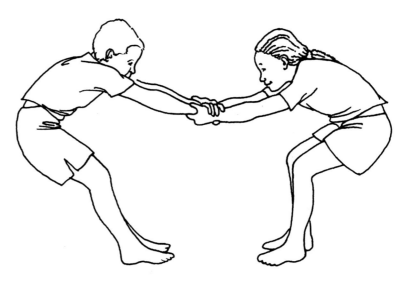

Hanging Bridge

"Find a partner who is about the same height as you are. Clasp your hands around the other person's wrists. Now both of you will lean back with straight legs. Take a breath together. Then sit down, breathing together. Then move into a squat together, pulling on each other to stretch out the upper back. Then slowly move up to standing and repeat."

j. Listen for Your Breath

"Sit tall in your seat and bring your hands to heart center. Close your eyes and listen for your own breath. After four breaths (a breath is a full inhale and a full exhale), open your eyes and you are ready to go home and enjoy the rest of your day!"

III. YOGA FROM TOP TO BOTTOM

I am my own laboratory.
—Lilias Folan

A Yoga Journey

The guided text in this section and the playful approach make it easy and fun to weave relaxation into any energizing practice. Focusing on meditative aspects of yoga as well as the release of tension during the poses may bring happy benefits to a yoga class. The yoking of doing and feeling in a variety of ways make the user-friendly scripts in this section widely adaptable to your group needs.

Many years ago, standing on a New York City bus during morning rush hour, I overheard an argument between two women who had accidentally bumped each other. Each was seized with the belief that it was the other's fault. One, who seemed to feel that the other woman was looking down on her, began proclaiming her mastery of yoga, and said she could bend her body all the way backwards. The other woman seemed to think she was crazy. The yoga practitioner turned to me for some reason, for support. Whatever I muttered, and I don't remember what it was, struck her deeply and she said, "You're saying you have to have a flexible mind, too, as well as a body." It seemed like a moment of enlightenment.

—Matthew Calhoun, New York City

A. For the Teacher: An Unexpected Gift

Teaching is a wonderful way to learn something. In my early 20's, I had a job in an after school program, creating learning projects for inner city children. After a few months of creating games and projects to teach reading, math, history, and whatever else seemed needed, I thought we might try yoga, which I learned from Lilias Folan's Public Television show, *Lilias, Yoga, and You!*

When I presented our first yoga project, *Be a Bridge!* my body was much more flexible than usual. The shift in my focus away from myself and my performance improved my performance—the first unexpected gift I received from sharing yoga.

At the end of our yoga session, the children lay on their mats, following my suggestions to imagine their bodies becoming so light they floated on a cloud, and then so heavy and relaxed, they were sinking into the ground. Deeply absorbed in our Final Relaxation, I expected we would enjoy the usual benefits of

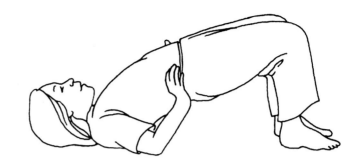

Bridge Pose

yogic peace. It was a different kind of relaxation we discovered, however: we rose full of a sunny excitement, recharged in an unexpected way. The yoga project caught on, and I began offering it once a week.

For the inexperienced teacher especially, you will want to get yoga "in your body" before teaching it. The scripts presented below can be molded to fit your needs. If you teach a script to yourself first and make it your own, you may discover how best to present it to others. Finding a live class, or working with a DVD such as *Lilias! Yoga 101 Workout for Beginners,* can be an exceptional way to reward yourself and in turn your students. Once you get the feel of something, new possibilities appear. When your body memorizes the idea behind the words, you can confidently mix and match, combine things in different ways, memorize parts, read verbatim, or wing it, using words and ideas that are more natural to you and your specific situation.

You can hold in mind a simple journey: a body moving through a progression of poses done on back, belly, sitting, all fours, standing, and flowing. This journey could be done in reverse, starting with Flow poses and ending with the Back to Earth section (keeping, of course, the Final Relaxation at the end.) Any part of this journey, such as "Magic Table Poses," could be done by itself.

When you teach yoga to children and teens, it may well surprise you with an unexpected reward. We cannot know in advance what this will be, but many times, when I was not thinking about it, or expecting it, or looking for it, in return for the care I took in offering the gift of yoga to children, something new and surprising was given to me.

Children learn through play.
—Socrates

B. Back to Earth: Poses Done on the Back

The first series of poses or *asanas* in our yoga journey help establish a good foundation for yoga practice. By drawing upon the relationship between the floor and the body, the deeper meaning of our ever-present relationship with the Earth is explored.

Notating breaths (one breath) in the text is a suggestion to leave a pause for the length of one full breath. Leaving breathing room for things to sink in more deeply can be a key part of successful yoga practice. If you do not go too fast, you may get to yoga more quickly!

1. Relaxation Pose: *Savasana*

Teacher: "You can lie down on your back, feet hip distance apart. Let your feet flop out, your arms a few inches from your side, palms pointed up. (One breath) And make sure your spine is in line with your chin, the top of your head. And now you have begun a very important yoga posture called *Savasana*, or Relaxation Pose.

And let's start at the bottom, because anything you do in life, everything you build, needs a good foundation. And feel the floor under your mat, holding you up, supporting you. (One breath) And feel how secure it is, how stable.

You don't see the foundation, holding up the building, but you can feel it's there. (One breath) You can notice that safe feeling you have when something powerful and safe is beneath you. (One breath)

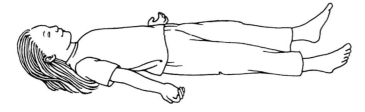

Relaxation

And we want to keep that safe, secure feeling as we work. Because we're going to build something: a practice of yoga that can be healthy and fun for you. And beneath this practice, is a feeling of caring, and safety. And simply by lying on your mat, which cushions and protects you, you can feel the floor, holding the mat, and the building and its foundation, safely supporting you, and beneath that, the whole earth. (One breath) And think about the earth, and let yourself daydream, anything you like, maybe trees growing, or sunshine, birds, water . . . (One breath) And you have made a wonderful beginning!"

2. Listening From Head to Toe

"And listen to the sounds outside yourself, and what do you hear? Are there sounds outside the room? Sounds inside the room? (One breath)

And let yourself hear the sound of your own breathing. What does it sound like, inside your head—breathing in, breathing out . . . (One breath)

And if you said something to your toes, do you think they would hear you? And can you wiggle the toes on your left foot? (Wiggle toes)

"And how does that feel, to ask your toes to do something, and have them do it for you? And sometimes there will be a conversation between your toes and your brain before you can even think. If you step on something that is too sharp,

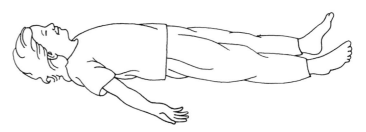

More Relaxation

your toes will tell you. They might say, "This hurts!" and the brain might say, "Move back." And in doing yoga, you may notice that you and your body listen to each other. And if something begins to hurt, your body is telling you to move away from it. And if your back is uncomfortable, you might hear it telling you that it needs to stop, or it needs to take a good stretch. And we want you to feel free to listen to your body, because it will teach you wonderful things." (One breath)

3. Both Sides (Side Stretches)

a. Right Side Stretch

"So let's play a game with a nice stretch, and with your eyes closed, without moving, find your right side. And take your time as you feel your right side—your right leg, right hip, right side of your chest, right shoulder, right arm, right ear . . . (One breath)

And then leaving the left side right where it is, you can stretch your right leg out, and push out with your heel as far as it will go. (One breath)

And now relax your leg and heel and let them go out a little further . . . (One breath) and move your right arm above your head and push the heel of the hand back as far as it will go . . . (One breath) and relax the shoulder and arm and let them stretch a little further . . . (One breath)

And focus on the air going in your right nostril . . . (One breath)

And move your right hand back to your side, by your thigh, and let your whole body relax . . . (One breath)

And notice your right side (One breath)

And find your left side (One breath)

And is there any difference?" (One breath)

b. Left Side Stretch

"And now in your mind's eyes, see your left side, and without moving it, just imagine it stretching: your left leg, left hip, left side of your chest, left arm, shoulder, fingers (Two breaths) And now, leaving the right side relaxing where it is, you can stretch your left side . . . (One breath)

And relax and let things go out a little further . . . (One breath)

And focus on the air moving and in out of your left nostril . . . (One breath)

And lower your left hand, and let your whole body relax . . . (One breath).

And notice your right side . . . (One breath) Left side . . . (One breath)

And notice both sides . . . (One breath)

And notice your breathing through both sides of your nose, and notice both sides of your body (One breath)

And it can be a wonderful thing to notice both sides. And they may be different, but in yoga, as in life, it is important to pay attention to both sides. And let's stretch out both sides at once, in any way you'd like, just give your whole body a nice stretch . . .

And bring your body back to *Savasana*, Relaxation Pose, arms at sides, palms up, feet flopped out to the side, spine, head, chin, and tailbone in a nice straight line . . . (One breath)

And you can lie still and relax for a minute and simply notice how your body feels, and see if it is getting more relaxed, at home, and comfortable." (One to three breaths)

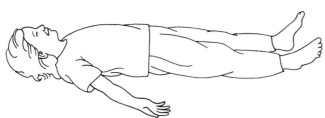

More Relaxation

114

4. Up and Down (Pelvic Tilt)

"And now, with your arms resting comfortably at your sides, palms up, slide your feet up towards your buttocks, soles of your feet flat on the ground, so your knees are up in the air. And settle your lower back into the floor so it's nice and flat against the mat, and gently push with the soles of the feet and the lower back, but let everything else be nice and relaxed . . . and then release, and let everything just relax. (Two breaths)

"And notice your belly button . . . and the muscles beneath there . . . push them down against the floor, and up towards your heart . . . so they are going down and up at the same time . . . down towards the floor, and up towards your heart . . . (One breath)

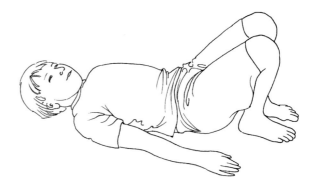

Up and Down

And let your neck and shoulders and arms be nice and relaxed . . . and if you need to move your neck a little to remind it that it doesn't have to be rigid and tense . . . that's fine. (One breath)

And remember this nice feeling behind your belly button of down and up at the same time . . . down towards the floor and up towards your heart . . ."

5. Leg Lifts

"And let those belly muscles relax and lift your legs . . . (Legs up)

And now notice your back pressing down against the floor as your legs are raised up . . . keep your arms and hands and shoulders nice and relaxed so all the pushing is with the belly muscles. (One breath)

And let your neck relax . . . then slowly lower your legs . . . and let your feet flop off to the side. (One breath)

And yoga is a joining of mind and body, so let's get your head in this and just IMAGINE that you're lifting your legs . . . and notice how your hips feel, and your stomach feels, as you imagine lifting your legs. (One breath)

Now, Yoga Leg Lifts begin with the muscles of the belly. So gently pull those muscles down to the floor and up towards

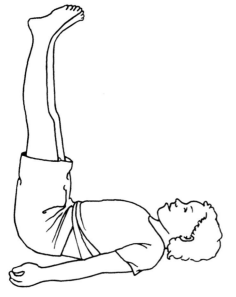

Leg Lifts

your heart . . . (One breath) Then let your belly relax and slowly and comfortably lift your legs up just a few inches . . . (Legs up and hold) and imagine a magic yoga magnet gently pulling on the bottoms of your feet, pulling your heels and gently stretching your legs out . . . notice your hip sockets (One breath) and then the magnet stops and you can slowly lower your legs to the floor. (Legs down)

And you can notice how your legs feel, resting comfortably against the floor, and how your body feels . . ." (One breath)

6. Both Sides II (Side Rolls)

a. Preparation for Side Rolls

"And now you can put your arms out like a 'T'—right arm out straight, left arm out straight, palms up, and place the soles of your feet flat on the floor, bending the knees. Slide your heels towards your buttocks, comfortably apart . . . roll your head to look out over your left arm . . . head straight so you can see the ceiling . . . head to look out over right arm . . . look up to see the ceiling . . . and now . . . seeing the ceiling . . . not moving your head

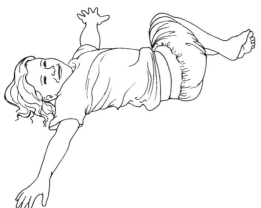

Side Rolls

. . . let your view expand so you can also see to the right and left . . . (One breath) This is called peripheral vision, and even if you don't remember that seeing to both sides is called peripheral vision, your eyes can still remember to have excellent peripheral vision and see both sides . . ."

b. Side Rolls

"And notice your belly button and the muscles behind it, and press them down to the ground . . . and up towards your heart . . . curl your knees up towards your chest . . . relax your belly . . . and keep your head where it is . . . looking straight up . . . roll your knees from side to side . . . under the left arm (knees roll to the left,) then under the right arm (knees roll to the right,) left, right . . . six times altogether . . . left, right, left right . . . left, right, left, right . . . back to center . . . now keeping the knees curled in towards the chest, without moving the knees, roll the head slowly left, right . . . left, right . . . left, right . . . back to center, place the soles of the feet on the mat, slide legs straight out, let feet flop to side, arms by side a few inches away from the body, palms up . . . and ask your body how it feels . . . And just notice that it tells you . . . how it feels . . . and take your time with this . . . and notice your breaths as well." (A few breaths)

7. Fish (*Matsyasana*)

a. Fish Meditation

"And there is a phrase, 'Like a fish out of water,' which means when you are not comfortable with your surroundings. And let's play a little game, and take in some air and hold your breath . . . and imagine, if you don't mind, a beautiful fish, but he's flopping around on a raft, floating on a beautiful lake. And he's really struggling to breathe and to get back into the water. And maybe sometimes you've felt a little like that—not being at home in your surroundings, and things were not going well. So let's give the fish a helping hand, and imagine that someone tilts the raft, and he slides right into the lake! And now he's swimming and he's a fish IN water. And let yourself breathe comfortably, (All let out breath) and notice all the good air all around you. And unlike a fish, you do very well breathing air."

b. Fish Pose *(Matsyasana)*

"And now, you can turn your palms over so they face down, and you can slide them into your back pockets (if you had them) for Fish Pose. (One breath). And notice your palms and forearms against the floor. (One breath)

And notice your breathing. And pushing with your palm and forearms, give your back a nice arch, from the very base of the spine, up towards the shoulders and push and pull yourself up into a nice arch, head off the floor . . . relax your neck and shoulders . . . and let yourself breathe shallowly. (Two breaths)

Fish Pose

And that is called "The Fish." And come out of it, very slowly, noticing how your spine moves, and come into *Savasana*, Relaxation Pose, arms a few inches from your sides, palms up, let your feet flop out, and notice your beautiful breathing."

8. Free Stretch (Coming out of *Savasana*)

"And now you can ask your body if it would like to stretch and if it wants to. Whenever you're ready, in any way you'd like, let your body stretch itself."

C. Belly Poses

Let us turn our attention to the belly. If you place your thumb on your navel with your palm sideways beneath your thumb, you will locate the abdominal muscle. This is the area to keep in mind when we use the word 'belly'.

Perhaps you can remember lying on your front in bed and enjoying a wonderful peaceful feeling in your stomach. The following games and exercises explore this central meeting place where you feel the sensations and emotions of being alive.

1. Belly Breathing

Teacher: "And now you can roll over onto your belly and you can make a pillow out of your hands and rest your head on the pillow. (One breath)

And notice your breathing against the floor. (One breath) It's very easy to feel where the air is, when it's pressing against the floor. And this can help you become more aware of your breathing. (One breath)

And now, breathe into your stomach, and notice how the air pressing against the floor lifts your stomach. (Inhale) And let the air go. (Exhale) And breathe in to your stomach and mid-section . . . (Inhale) And notice the air pressing against the floor and lifting this area. And let the air go. (Exhale)

And breathe in to your stomach, mid-section and chest.

And notice the air pressing against the floor and lifting your chest. (Inhale)

And let the air go." (Exhale and one more breath)

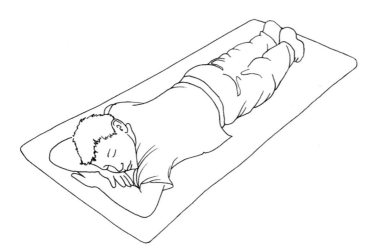

Belly Breathing

118

2. Belly Laughing

"And now breathe in air into your stomach. (Inhale)

And laugh from your stomach: 'Ho ho ho' as you let out the air.

OK, and now breathe into your stomach and mid-section. (Inhale)

And laugh from your mid-section, 'Ho ho ho,' as you let out the air.

And breathe in through your stomach and mid-section and chest. (Inhale)

And laugh from your chest as you let out the air: 'Ho ho ho!'

And laughing from your belly can sound different from another area. Maybe the laughter is higher from the chest. Try laughing from your belly and then your chest. And then notice how the sound might change."

(All experiment with "Ho ho ho's")

Note: The sounds "Ho ho ho" may lead to spontaneous laughter. Laughing is a wonderful massage for the inner organs and has been associated with physiological healing and health.

3. Belly Smile

(With grateful acknowledgement to the inspiration of Lilias Folan's teaching of the "Yoga Smile". For examples, see, *Inner Smile Relaxation*; *Lilias! Yoga Gets Better with Age*, Rodale Inc., 2005, p. 12; and the CD *The Inner Smile*).

"And now let's try a different kind of smile. Some smiles shine outside yourself, and some can shine inside. So imagine a warm, sunny smile—have that feeling of the corners of your lips going up . . . and let that smiling, sunny feeling travel to the back of your mouth, and feel the hollow in the back of your mouth become more open, and relaxed, as the smiling warmth fills it . . . (One breath)

And let the feeling of the warmth and sunshine of the smile move deeper in, down your throat, relaxing your neck . . . (One breath)

into your chest . . . (One breath)

and down beneath your ribs, into your back, your lungs, your stomach . . . filling it with healing warmth and relaxation . . . (One breath)

And smile down into your lungs . . . let that smile move from inside your mouth down all the way to the bottom of your lungs, and if there is any dark place down there that needs warming up, just feel the smile spreading even deeper . . . (One breath)

And this is the "Yoga Smile". And you can give yourself a nice yoga smile whenever you like. All you have to do is remember that yoga works from the inside out and also from the outside in. So you can smile down inside yourself. And whenever part of you might feel sad, or tired, or confused, or upset, or tense . . . you can notice this big smile starting inside your mouth, and let it shine down inside you . . . (One breath)

And let's try an experiment. Let that smile go up into your brain . . . and see if you feel it smile back." (Two breaths)

4. Caterpillar

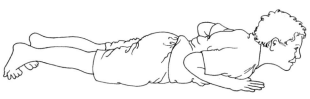

Caterpillar

"OK, and now feel your breathing, going in your stomach, mid-section, and chest . . . And going out . . . And going in . . . And going out. And as you continue to breathe in this beautiful way, think of a caterpillar on a warm, sunny, relaxing day . . . (One breath)

And this caterpillar may not be going fast, but still has that feeling of going somewhere wonderful! And move your elbows by your chest, palms down, fingers pointed forward, by the sides of your head. And curl your toes under, as if you were going to use them to push yourself forward. (One breath)

And now, staying in one place, push with your toes so your spine moves forward. Your body as a whole stays where it is, but your spine stretches forward. (Spine elongates forward)

And now, push against the ground with your forearms to pull your spine back. (Spine elongates backwards)

And use your toes and arms to move your spine forward, so your spine is going forward. (Spine elongates forward)

And use your elbows and forearms to move your spine back. (Spine elongates backwards) And do this once more, at your own pace, in your own way, comfortably moving your spine forward and back . . ."

5. Caterpillar Walk

"And now, if you don't mind, imagine you're a caterpillar on a beautiful day moving along, and you may not know where you're going, but you're feeling happy and you have the feeling you're going somewhere wonderful!

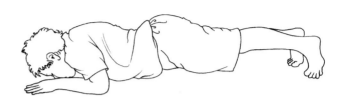

Caterpillar Walk

(One breath) And move yourself forward on your belly in any way you like. And we'll call this the caterpillar walk. Move forward in a comfortable way . . . and any way you do it is the way *this* caterpillar moves! And then you can move back to where you started. And remember the feeling: you are going somewhere wonderful!"

6. Cobra (*Bhujangasana*)

"And now we're going to do a yoga exercise called Cobra, and this is very good for the bones in your spine. A cobra is a powerful snake, and practicing this exercise can keep your spine powerful and strong and flexible. So now, you can place your palms flat on the floor beneath shoulders, fingers close together, elbows up, close to your chest, and rest your forehead and nose on the ground. Move

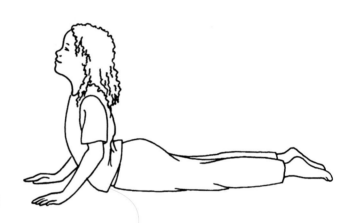

Cobra

your feet together, your toes out straight, nice and relaxed, and we're going to slowly uncoil. You can slowly move your chin away from your chest, so your nose and chin brush against your mat as you slowly bend the neck and head backward, keeping the chest close to the ground . . . (One breath)

And let the power come from the hips and spine, so just use your hands for balance, not to push too hard. And breathing in, slowly raise your head, shoulders, chest and upper abdomen, up to the belly button, above the ground, arching back, chin up in a nice arch. (One breath)

And let the tongue shoot out a couple times and then relax your jaw . . . and let the neck and shoulders and back relax . . . so the head can maybe stretch back a little more. (Head back further)

And you can feel the floor pushing into your hands, and your hands pushing back into the floor, and the pelvic area, between your hips, against the floor, and you can use this pressure to help support the cobra . . . (One breath)

And you can release and return slowly to the starting position in reverse order, slowly coiling up, chin, nose, and forehead to the mat. And rest comfortably, and notice how your back and spine and hips feel. (One breath)

And think about all the places in your body where there are bones. These bones are alive, just like you are. Throughout your life, these bones will be growing. Even when you're grown up, little cells like jackhammers will be getting rid of old bone and other little cells will be growing new bone. Every three years or so, you will have an entirely new set of bones. And if you feel like it, you can practice the Cobra again, or you can rest a little while longer." (Leave time for optional repeat of Cobra)

7. Half Locust (*Ardha Salabhasana*)

a. Preparation for Half Locust

(Lying on front)

"And you can make a pillow out of your hands, and we're going to learn a yoga pose called "The Half Locust." Yoga poses can bring relief to your body in a number of ways by preventing problems that might develop later. The Half Locust can send extra blood to nourish your inner organs and heart and brain. And your belly is an inner organ, and can you notice your inner organs, inside you, resting comfortably against the mat? (One breath)

And notice where your heart is, inside the left side of your chest . . . (One breath)

And notice where your brain is, protected inside your skull." (One breath)

b. Half Locust (*Ardha Salabhasana*)

"And to do the Half Locust, lying face down on your mat, place your hands at your sides by your thighs, palms up. Please keep your feet together, and your chin on the floor. Gently press your right hip area into the mat, and breathe in as you lift up your left leg. As you lift your LEFT leg, pay close attention to your RIGHT leg. (When the left leg is lifted)

And you can relax a bit, and push with your forearms and the backs of your hands as you raise your left leg even higher. Feel the arch from the lower spine all the way up. Slowly, in slow motion, lower your left leg. (When leg is lowered)

And that's the Half Locust on the left side! And now, lying here comfortably, without doing anything yet, think about doing the Half Locust on the other side. And notice your left leg. And how would your body move if you wanted to lift the right leg for Half Locust? (One breath) And now you can try it on your own, the Half Locust, raising the right leg."

Challenge: Full Locust
(Students are lying face down, arms at sides, palms up.)
In preparation for Full Locust, drawing the attention to the backs of the hands (which will be used along with the forearms to push up) is an interesting exercise in awareness. When you know something really well, you might say, "I know this like the back of my hand."

"And let's see how the backs of your hands will help you do a Full Locust. So your hands are at your side, palms up, so the backs of your hands are against the mat. And you can make loose fists, and slide them so that the pinkies go under the rim of your hips, and the thumb part goes on the mat. (Slide fists under the hips)

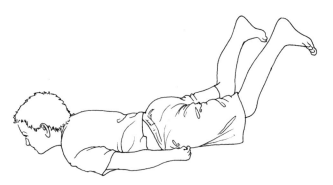

Full Locust

And feel them against the mat, against the floor. And maybe you can feel support from way below, from the ground underneath the building . . . . (One breath)

And keep your legs snuggled close together and your knees straight and take a nice breath and hold. And now imagine magic threads around your ankles, and they lift your legs up. You can help by using the muscles behind your belly button to help lift, and push with your forearms and the backs of your hands, drawing your elbows in. (One breath)

And keeping your head down, this is the Locust Pose. When the locust bends its head to eat and raises its tail, it looks exactly like you do, now! Well, maybe not exactly . . . and you can let out your breath, and slowly lower the legs to the floor without bending your knees.

And this will help your lungs and chest become healthy and strong. It can strengthen muscles in the lower back, the abdomen, and straighten out the base of the spine. And notice how you feel inside yourself, in your belly, and see how your lower spine feels, your lower back, your legs, thighs, hips, and your wrists. And the backs of your hands. (One breath) And maybe you can notice how nice it is to be noticed, sometimes."

8. Treasure Boat Story

"And now you can make a pillow out of your hands and I'll tell you a little story, so you can rest before we do the next pose.
Two people with good, little boats went to an island where there was a lot of treasure. The seas were rough, but the boats had no problem getting to the island. The first sailor loaded his boat with treasure, ten times more than he weighed. When he set off, out in the open seas, the waves were big. The treasure slid to one side of the boat pulling that side out-of-balance and down low in the water. The sea rushed into the boat and it sank.
The second boat coming from the island saved the first sailor, although his boat and treasure were lost. 'Why doesn't your boat sink in these rough seas?' asked the poor sailor. 'I knew my boat could carry two or three people, so I took my body weight in treasure and no more,' said the rich sailor."

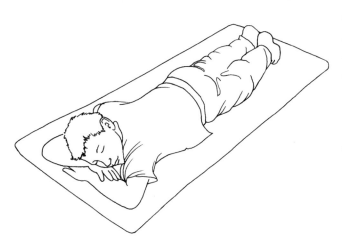

Listening

9. The Boat Pose

"And now we're going to do a pose called The Boat. And this is a wonderful pose to teach you balance. So you can stretch your arms forward on both sides of your head with your palms turned down. And keep your forehead face down on the mat. And put your feet and legs together, so they kind of snuggle together against your body.
And now, press your arms and legs firmly against the floor in a balanced way And your forehead, too, but not so it hurts. Notice if one leg or arm isn't pressing and press that one, too, so all is even and firm.
And relax and release, and let your body just float on your breathing. (Two breaths) Imagine that magic strings are lifting your ankles and wrists, and raise your arms, head, neck, shoulders, and feet and legs all together, in a balanced way.

Keep your upper arms close to your ears and your feet together. And get a nice, balanced stretch, so your body is curved from the fingers to the toes, and they are level with each other.

Pause, and see if you want the strings to lift you up just a little higher. But remember, only go as high as you need to go to. And stay nice and balanced on the lower part of your belly, which is the only part touching the ground.

Now, this is called The Boat Pose, and when you do it, you breathe life into it and it breathes more life into you. And now slowly and evenly lower the arms, legs, head . . . and you can make a pillow of your hands and rest. (One breath) And let yourself float on your breathing, as if you're a boat, and remember, your body is a treasure you will have your whole life. (One breath)

And notice your breathing against the floor, and have you noticed how great it is to rest after you work at something? Work makes rest better, and rest makes work better. If you do too much of either, the fun might go out of it." (Two breaths)

Note: When you return to Boat Pose in the future, you might ask the students if they remember the story of the boat with the treasure. Perhaps in retelling it they will change it, which can be a lovely way to engage their imaginations.

D. Sitting Poses: Taking Notice

As we continue our Yoga Journey, we can "sit up and take notice" of how to direct attention in a helpful way. Instead of saying, "Everybody listen to me," a yoga teacher can direct a child's mind to its body. "OK, everyone, now we're going to play a listening game!" It might go like this . . .

1. Listening Meditation
Teacher: "Sitting on your mat in any way you'd like, you can listen to your body and see what it might be telling you . . . (One breath)

And maybe your body wants to . . . (One breath)
shift somehow, to become more comfortable . . . (One breath)

And maybe some part is telling you that it's more tense than it needs to be right now . . . (One breath) and you can relax . . . (One breath)

And you can listen to your breathing . . . (One breath)

And it makes a sound, a soft sound, and maybe your jaw is more tense that it needs to be, and you could . . . (One breath) well, maybe your body wants to move, maybe it wants to stretch a little, or move in a way you don't expect . . . There are a thousand ways to sit, and just let your body move in any way it likes. Staying in a sitting position, just move your body in any way you would like to . . . (Two or three breaths)

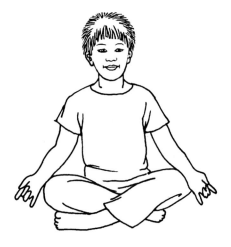

Now, as we do more yoga, you can keep listening to your body and what it's telling you.

And if it ever tells you that something is causing you pain, just don't go there. We want stretch, but pain is your body's way of telling you to stop . . . (One breath)

And sometimes your body begins to feel overloaded, like it has had enough for a little while, and you can stop and rest." (One breath)

And as we learn to listen to our bodies during yoga, it can help you: learn to concentrate. Learn to focus. Learn to listen. Learn to work to please yourself. And think how much easier your life will be when you learn these things!" (One breath)

Listening meditation

Note: Sometimes verbal suggestions knock around for awhile in the back of the mind, follow their own pathways, and come out in a beautiful place. You might say the magic words, "Maybe your body wants to move, maybe it wants to stretch a little, or move in a way you don't expect . . . and just let your body move in any way it likes," and around 10 or 15 minutes later, someone might find the delightful desire to have a nice stretch in a wonderful, liberating, yogic kind of way, without forcing, full of release.

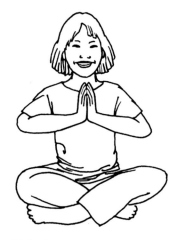

Listening meditation

Things you do and say now with children may register later . . . so do not be disheartened if you feel you are not being heard, or not getting through as fully as you would like. There is an unconscious listening mind as well as a conscious one, and sometimes allowing time for the unconscious to do its part is a learning body's best friend.

2. Butterfly Pose *(Baddha Konasana)*

"And now, we're going to warm up your legs for the Butterfly Exercise. So you can move your legs out in front of you, and point your toes up towards the ceiling. (One breath) And why don't you rub your left knee, a nice warm rub to warm it up, and squeeze it and massage it in a supportive way. (Massage knee)

And the right knee. (Massage right knee) And with your legs out straight, your toes up towards the ceiling, you can move your arms out over your legs, so your palms are pointed down. And notice your knees. (One breath)

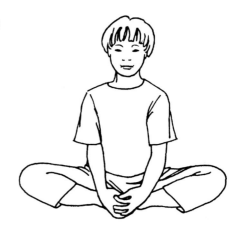

Butterfly

What kind of sound would they make if you tapped them up and down on the floor? Let's try it. (All move knees up and down, listening to the sound it makes.) And let them rest, and notice your legs against the floor. Do they feel more flat against the floor, as those muscles relax? (One breath)

And now, bring the soles of your feet together, and you can hold your feet with your hands, your fingers over the tops, and your thumbs on the bottoms. And you can rub the soles of your feet with your thumbs. You can press them, and work out some tension. (Foot massage) And now, holding on to your feet, move your knees up and down, like wings flapping . . . Knees move up and down)

And rest, and notice your hip joints . . . (One breath)
They're getting a nice work out, aren't they?

And if you want to, you can move your feet a little closer in towards your hips, and flap again, moving your knees up and down, like a butterfly's wings flapping. (Knees move up and down)

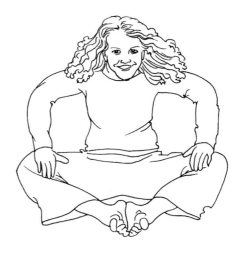

Butterfly

And as you do this, you can shut your eyes and maybe you'll see a butterfly . . . or a field of butterflies . . . (More flapping) a butterfly landing on a rock. (More flapping)

But whatever you see, let your legs become still and notice your body. (One breath)

And notice your hip joints . . . the blood flowing through them . . . the warmth."

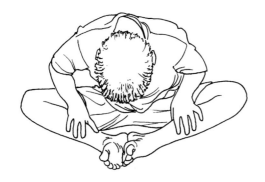

Star Pose

3. Star Pose

"And the Butterfly is a good warm-up for Star Pose. So with your feet together in Butterfly Position, look up to the ceiling, and way up above to where the stars are. And notice how your spine opens up, and arch your chest up, gently lifting it and making more room inside your ribs, as you move your head back . . . (One breath)

And now bend forward, your head going out over your lap towards your feet, and your elbows out over your knees. Slide your knees out a little if you need to. You can make a star with your elbows and knees and head being the point . . . (One breath)

And imagine a sky full of stars and they're smiling down on you and touching your muscles with loving, relaxing magic . . . (One breath)

And come back to Butterfly Pose, with your back straight, and you can arch your spine again, lifting your chest up. And you're moving it in the opposite direction from when you bent over, to give it a lot of good possibilities . . ." (One breath)

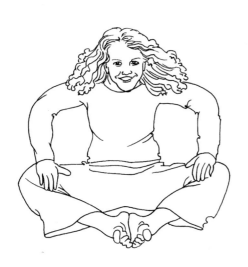

Butterfly

And now you can turn your torso a little right and hold your knees with your hands and bend down over your right knee. And notice your breathing . . . (One breath)

And come back to Butterfly position, and gently arch your back, and lift your chest upward, and make a lot of nice room inside your ribs. And maybe you can kind of feel them spread out a little, and notice your breathing, going in and out . . . (One breath)

And you can turn your torso left and hold your left knee and calf and bend down over your left knee, now, and just RELAX into it. This isn't about working hard and pushing and being tense, it's about letting go and just kind of flopping, and let your chest and head kind of rest . . . (One breath)

And back to Butterfly Pose. Nice arch up . . . (One breath) And back to Star Pose, where you bend forward, elbows out over your knees, and make a nice, five pointed star, pulling your tailbone back." (One breath)

4. Merry-Go-Round

"Have you ever seen a Merry-go-round turning round? It goes very smoothly and evenly, and now just circle your head to the left moving your arms and hands with them so your chest is over your left knee, in a smooth circle, not too fast . . . (Circle left)

And keep circling back . . . (Circle back)

And to the right, back over the right knee . . . (Circle right)

And forward, into Star Position, and another go-round, left . . ." (Circle left)

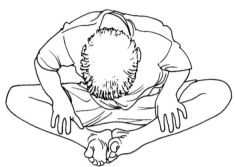

Star Pose

Back . . . (Circle back) . . . Right . . . (Circle right)

And back to Star Position, forward . . . (One breath) . . . And now reverse direction, and go to the right . . . (Circle right) . . . and back . . . (Circle back) And to the left . . . (Circle left) . . . And forward . . . (Circle forward) And one more go-round . . . (Circle 360 degrees) . . . and back to sitting, in Butterfly Position . . . (One breath)

And notice your hip joints, and just let them relax, and pull your feet towards you and then flap your butterfly wings one more time! (All flap together)

And see if your knees go down more easily now. Remember how it was at first, and see if they've loosened up." (More flapping)

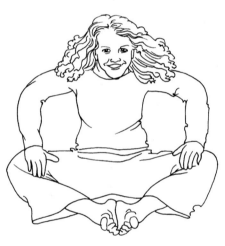

Butterfly

5. Putting It All Together

"So now, we can put all this together, Butterfly Warm-up, Butterfly, Star, and Merry-Go-Round. And let's try a little poem, to help us remember. So you can put your legs out straight in front of you, toes pointed up, and

Move your knees, up and down
With a flappy happy sound . . . (Knees move up and down)
And now Butterfly position Flap your knees, Butterfly
Wonder where you'll go today? (Butterfly flapping)
And for Star Pose, Arch your back, gentle now
Elbows on your shins curl down . . .

Arch your back, stretch it freeeeeeee . . . (One breath)
Curl it down towards your left knee.

Arch your back happily
Curl it down towards your right knee.

Arch your back, gentle now
Elbows on your shins, curl down . . .

From your hips go around
Move like a Merry-go-round
Other way, turn around
Like a smooth Merry go round

Flap your knees Butterfly
Wonder where you'll land today?

And you can roll on back to the ground for relaxation."

6. Butterfly Relaxation

"And let your feet flop over to the side, arms a few inches away from your body, palms up . . . and notice your heart. See if you can feel it beating in your chest . . . (One breath) And while you are resting and letting your body absorb all the good stretching and moving and learning. (One breath)

There's a butterfly flitting by, black and orange with little flecks of white, a Monarch butterfly, flying around, here and there . . . maybe more than one, and sometimes your thoughts are like that. You can watch them, flying here, landing there, trying this out, flying around, exploring . . . and the butterfly lands on your nose . . . don't move a muscle, but see if you can feel . . . (One breath) and it flies off. And did you know a Monarch butterfly can travel all the way from Canada to Mexico? Over 1,800 miles. They are powerful travelers, and they will go very far. So delicate, but they have the power to migrate over a thousand miles . . . (One breath)

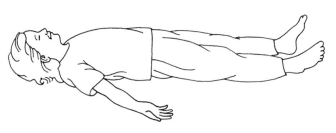

Butterfly Relaxation

And just notice your thoughts, and images flowing through your mind, and notice how time is passing—is it fast or slow? (One breath)

And feel your breathing . . . your body resting against the floor . . . (One breath)

And when you're ready, you can sit up, and we're going to the Spinal Twist."

7. Spinal Twist

"And can you reach behind your back with your hands and feel your spine? And see if you can feel two or three joints, between the little sections of the spine called vertebrae. (Feel behind back)

And see how much of your spine you can touch and feel. You can use your thumbs, the knuckles, both hands . . ." (Explore spine with hands. Ask questions about what the spine is like. Bring out that it is both hard and protective, but also very flexible. It can bend and turn in six different directions.)

a. Right Spinal Twist

"And now let's do a nice twist to keep your spine strong and flexible. You can sit cross-legged, with your right leg folded over your left . . . (One breath)

And place your left palm against your left thigh. And place your right palm on your left knee and give it a nice, friendly rub . . . (Rub the knee)

And now, twist your spine to the left, pushing gently with your right hand against your knee, chin looking over left shoulder . . . head turned to the left. Eyes looking as far to the left as they can. And what are you seeing? Do you notice what you're seeing? (One breath) And now, moving only your eyes, nothing else, move your eyes to the right!

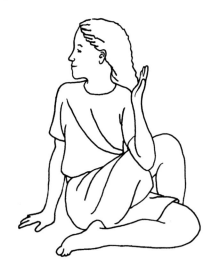

Seated Twist

(Eyes shift right) And what are you seeing? Just take a moment to notice for yourself . . . (One breath)

And now, moving only your neck and head, move your neck and head to the right, in a smooth, easy way . . . and relax your right shoulder and look over your right shoulder, as far as you can . . . but without moving your spine . . . (Neck and head to the right)

And now let your spine follow and swing around way to the right, and put your left palm against your right knee and your hand on the ground behind you . . . thumb pointed into the middle of the back and gently stretch everything to the right . . . so you're looking over your right shoulder . . . (One breath) and come back to center . . . (One breath)

And in yoga, if we bend one way, we then want to bend the opposite way to keep the body and mind in balance. So let's do the other side."

(Instructions in reverse for Left Spinal Twist follow for your reference:)

"Fold your left leg over your right . . . (One breath)
Place your right palm against your right thigh. Place your left palm on your right knee and rub the knee. Twist spine to the right, pushing with your left hand against your knee, chin over right shoulder. Head turned to the right. Eyes looking as far to the right as they can. (One breath)

Moving only your eyes, move eyes to the left. (One breath.) Moving only neck and head, move neck and head to the left . . . relax left shoulder and look over your left shoulder, as far as you can . . . but without moving your spine. (Neck and head to the left)

Let spine follow and swing around way to the left, and put right palm against left knee and left hand on the ground behind you . . . thumb pointed into the middle of the back and gently stretch everything to the left . . . so you're looking over your left shoulder . . . (One breath) and come back to center."

E. Magic Table Poses

1. Magic Table Pose

Here is a playful game utilizing an imaginary ball to help children develop body control, awareness, and appreciation.

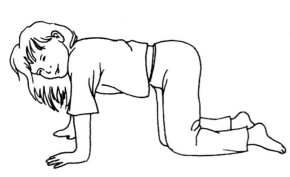

Flat table pose

"Now we're going to find out about a magic table, which has a special present for you. It will be fun to play with, but will also help you . . . (One breath)

So, let yourself be like a table, on all fours, with your back nice and straight. Let your back be level with the floor, with your hands and knees making a stable and secure rectangle under the table. Make your hands and knees nice and even, and your back flat above them . . . (One breath)

Imagine there is a kind of ball of light and energy on your back . . . (One breath) Gently tilt up your chest just a little bit . . . and pretend the ball is slowly rolling down your back, getting bigger, making it feel good . . . (One breath)

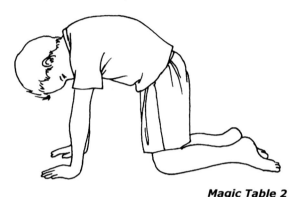

Magic Table 1

Magic Table 2

Gently and slowly raise your hips and lower your chest so the ball rolls from your lower back to the middle of your back . . . (One breath) . . . and then between your shoulders, gently touching your neck . . . bringing wonderful feeling to wherever it touches. And it sticks to your neck until you tilt back, higher now . . . and it slowly rolls back down between your shoulders, your middle back, lower back, as you arch your spine . . . lifting your head up and tailbone up in a nice . . . gentle stretch . . . and it sticks to your tailbone . . . and as you gently stretch, it sends good, relaxing, healing, loving energy right up your spine and around your rib cage to the front . . . and wherever it needs to go to help you . . . feel wonderful! (Two breaths). And back to a flat Table Pose . . . (One breath)

And notice your hands and knees in a nice rectangle, back flat and level . . . and the magic ball of light and energy is sinking into your hips and legs . . . knees . . . calves . . . feet . . . like a big blob of healing energy . . . changing size and shape to just fit inside your body . . . and relax your elbows . . . straight, but not locked . . . and as you breathe . . . and notice your breathing . . . notice how the breath gets bigger inside you as it comes in . . . like it's filling a sack in your lungs, stomach and chest . . . and how the sack gets smaller on the way out . . . (One breath) . . . and your body gently and magically changes size and shape as you breathe . . . easily . . . naturally . . ."

2. Yoga Eyes

a. Looking Behind

"Begin in Table Pose. What if you wanted to see what is behind you? Because, no matter where you're looking, whether you look through a microscope and see very small things, or a telescope and see very far things, or through your eyes and see very naturally . . . (One breath) . . . there'll always be more to see! You'll never have seen it all! And this keeps life interesting . . .

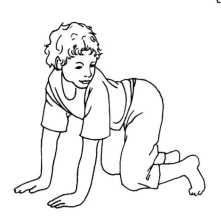

Yoga Eyes

So you might, keeping your knees and hands in a nice relaxed, secure base, slowly look around over your left shoulder and see what's back there. And go slowly so you can see how your spine stretches and grows longer and changes shape to allow your neck and head and eyes to move and see what's back there. (When head is looking over left shoulder, allow one more breath) And come forward to base position and look forward and just notice what you see. And does it look a little different now? Is it a new view of things?"

b. Looking Inside

"And shut your eyes and see your breathing traveling in and out . . . and notice how your belly and mid-section and chest rise and change shape as it goes in, and out . . . (One breath) . . . with its relaxing, nourishing, healing energy . . . (One breath) . . . and notice your nose . . . and does it change shape at all as the air passes in and out? Maybe a little? So little you barely notice?"

c. Looking Right

"And you can open your eyes . . . and notice how, whenever you open them, they simply see . . . on their own. These magic balls of energy and light are a great gift to you. They blink, and what if you looked over your right shoulder and behind you, to see what you could see? And go slowly, so you can see all the scenery on the way! And notice how your hips and spine move . . . and shut your eyes and notice if your hands and knees are pushing evening on the floor . . . And keep your neck relaxed and notice if the floor is pushing evenly against your hands and knees . . . and you can open your eyes again and swing your eyes forward."
(One breath)

d. Looking Under

"And slowly curl (up) your spine and let your head lower and look down at the floor and between your legs and behind you . . . lifting up your hips and lower back just a little . . . and then you can let the top of your head rest flat against the floor . . . right between your hands . . . and you can see behind you . . . and shut your eyes and notice the blood moving into

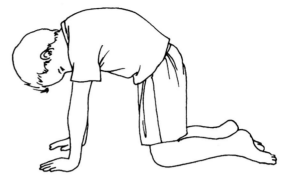

Looking Under

your head . . . that is very nice for your brain . . . and notice your breathing . . . and how you can breathe in whatever position you're in . . . (One breath) . . . And then open your eyes . . . come back to base . . . Magic Table Pose . . . and let your spine extend back a little . . . just naturally stretch out."

3. Down Dog Pose (*Adho mukha svanasana*)

"Find your Table Pose again. Imagine a dog is about to have a good stretch. Have you ever seen a dog or a cat stretch itself? There are many ways to stretch yourself . . . (One breath) . . . And dogs are known as being faithful, loyal, protective, playful—your dog will always love you, no matter what. So, let's say . . . your body is like a dog, and we're going to do a yoga stretch called "Downward Facing Dog."

To warm up, move your hips from side to side, and come back to Table Pose. Have you ever heard a dog moan sadly? Dogs are wonderful at letting it out . . . and sometimes a nice moan is a good way to get rid of some sadness . . . So let's all moan, a nice dog moan: 'aooooooo. . . .' (If the moaning leads to laughter, that's fine, because sometimes when you let out some sadness you discover some laughter . . .)

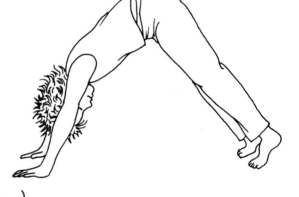

Down Dog

And now refocus on your hands and knees, even, stable, secure and spread your fingers out like stars . . . (One breath)

And point your face towards the floor, and turn your toes under, pushing off against the mat. And push with your hands onto the floor . . . lift the knees . . . legs straight, but not stiff . . . head between upper arms . . . lengthen spine . . . hips back . . . heels down a bit . . . nice stretch throughout back, legs, arms, fingers . . . head between the arms, looking down at the hands, and a nice dog moan! And a HAPPY dog moan! And lower the knees to the mat, and come back to Table Pose."

4. Magic Table Pose 2 ("Get Off My Back!")

This is a variant on the healing ball rolling up and down the spine. It allows children to use "negative" energy in a useful way.

"And let's pretend that someone has put a different kind of ball sitting on your back, and this ball isn't so nice. It's tiring and kind of heavy. It's not that happy, and makes you feel kind of tense. And someone has put this on your back . . . (One breath)

And sometimes people put things on a perfectly good table that don't belong there. And there's a wonderful phrase you can say to yourself, 'Get off my back!' Can you all say it with me? (All say "Get off my back!")

And gently come up to your knees, back straight, arms hanging down . . . pretend your back is very slippery and . . . (One breath) . . . whatever it was has rolled off your back, hit the ground somewhere, and popped like a soap bubble . . ." (One breath)

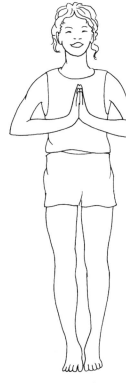

F. Stand Your Ground (*Tadasana*)

Tadasana, the Sacred Mountain Pose, provides a good starting point for all standing poses. To stand up is one thing. To more fully appreciate the art of standing is a gift of yoga.

1. Sacred Mountain Poem ("*Tadasana*")

"OK, let's all stand up as tall as is comfortable, feet hip-width apart. And we're going to act out a little poem that can help you learn a powerful yoga pose called *Tadasana*, or The Sacred Mountain Pose.

Stand with me and you will find
The power of a gentle mind.
(Teacher moves palms together as class follows)
Place each palm against each palm
And let them keep each other calm . . . (One breath)
Let your knees be straight but not
Tense, and feel them a lot . . . (One breath)

Sacred Mountain

136

Behind your belly button move
The muscles back, and up with love.

(Note: This is the pelvic tilt, practiced during the Back to Earth
    section.)
A mountain breeze may reach the town;
Ease your shoulders back and down . . . .(One breath)
Lasting as a mountain pine
Grows towards the sky, align your spine
And chin and head and heart and soul;
Accept the things you can't control . . . .(One breath) (Teacher
    moves thumb knuckles into indentation in the breastbone)
Move the knuckles of your thumbs
Against the place beneath your chest
That we may call the Lake of Rest
And love your heartbeat as it comes . . . (One breath)
This is called *Tadasana*, the Mountain Pose, the Strength of
    Calm.
Say with me, *Tadasana* (All say *Tadasana*)
Allow your head to slowly bow
As far as comfort will allow.
Stay with me, *Tadasana*,
The Sacred Mountain, strong and calm." (Two breaths)

2. Find Your Inner Sun (A Standing Meditation)

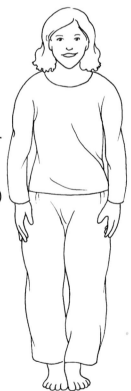

Mountain Pose

"And staying in *Tadasana*, you can lift your head so you're
looking forward, and notice what you see . . . (One breath)

And notice how your eyes feel—the physical feeling in your
eyes . . . (One breath)

And then bring your attention to your nose.

And notice the air moving in and out of it . . . (One breath)

And you don't have to change it, or stop it from changing,
simply notice it . . . (One breath)

You don't have to make yourself breathe in a relaxed
fashion, or stop yourself from breathing in a relaxed fashion,
simply notice your breathing, the flow of air, in, out . . . (One
breath)

And you might notice that it's a bit cool going in . . . (One
breath)

And you might notice that's it's warmer going out . . .
(One breath)

Cool going in, warm going out . . . (One breath)

And what do you suppose makes it warm? Well, it's you, of course. You have a body temperature—warmth, within yourself. There's a sun warming us from outside, keeping the world warm, and there's also a kind of mysterious sun of life within you, keeping you warm from the inside . . . (One breath)

And notice that warm air, going out, and cool, going in, and remember, something is warming that air, and that something is you . . . (One breath)

3. Walking Down the Mountain

"From your Mountain Pose, you can bow your head . . . and imagine a cliff covered with a sheet of ice . . . and at the bottom of the cliff is a lake that needs water . . . and Spring is coming . . . the sun's coming out and melting the ice . . . (One breath)

And pretend your arms have been frozen, but they are nice and thawed out . . . (One breath)

The ice, the stiffness has melted and gently let your arms drop, and dangle . . . (One breath)
and notice your breathing, in, out . . . (One breath)

And pretend that your arms have been tense, but tension is just flowing out your fingers (One breath) and water, melting ice, is flowing into the lake at your feet . . . (One breath)
and let any tension in your neck melt . . . (One breath)

Like warm sunshine melting ice, and your spine
. . . relax . . . let tension melt away, as your chin lowers to your chest . . . (One breath) . . . and as your spine slowly bends, touch your thighs with your middle fingers and let your middle and index fingers walk down your legs, inch by inch, little step by little step . . . knees, calves . . . spine loose, comfortable . . . notice your breathing, nothing is forced . . . if you need to, loosen your knees . . . and . . . look between your arms, and between your feet . . . and see how far down you want to go . . . maybe you want to touch your ankles, or your feet, or the ground, but stay comfortable, relaxed . . . feeling good, not forcing . . . breathing in, out . . . (One breath) and then slowly, inch by inch, smoothly let yourself rise up, noticing your breathing, each separate vertebra, arms dangle at your side, chin up, eyes looking straight forward . . . and what do you see? Does it look different than when you began?"

4. Mountain Pose

In this version, only some of the words of the Sacred Mountain Poem are used. If the poem has been done earlier, the echo of the unspoken words may guide the body deeper into the meaning of the posture.

"And back into *Tadasana*, the Sacred Mountain Pose, feet hip width apart, place each palm against each palm . . . (One breath)
Let your knees be straight but not tense . . . (One breath)
Behind your belly button move
The muscles back, and up . . . (One breath)
Ease your shoulders back and down . . . (One breath)
Align your spine
And chin and head and . . . (One breath).
(Teacher moves thumb knuckles into indentation in the breastbone)
Move the knuckles of your thumbs
Against the place beneath your chest . . . " (One breath)

5. Sacred Cow

(Similar to "Walking Down the Mountain," but now the fingers are not used as "training wheels" on the way down.)

"This next pose is called "The Cow". The people in India who developed yoga believe that cows were sacred. The Egyptians believed that cats were sacred. And when something is sacred, it is valuable and important and we treat it with great respect. And many people believe that within you is a little spark of something sacred.

So slowly, let your head lower, chin to chest, as your spine bends . . . arms dangle, loose, relaxed, inch by inch, slowly, fluidly, smoothly, and notice your breath, in, out, tension melting, you can just let your spine bend, and your arms dangle . . . and look between your arms, and between your feet . . . and see how far down you want to go . . . maybe you want to touch your ankles, or your feet, or the ground, but stay comfortable, relaxed . . . feeling good, not forcing . . . breathing in, out . . . (One breath)

And if you like you can bend your knees, and then straighten them again, and relax them, and see if you go down further . . . (One breath)

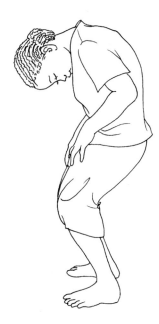

Sacred Cow

And you might try this again if you like, bend your knees, and then straighten them, let them relax, and see if you go down any further . . . (One breath)

and then slowly, inch by inch, smoothly let yourself rise up, noticing your breathing, each separate vertebra, arms dangle at your side, chin up, eyes looking straight forward . . .

(All slowly rise) and shut your eyes, and think about a lake . . . full of blue, happy water, now, summer has come, maybe people are swimming, splashing, having fun . . .

6. Free Style

Maturity is understanding
that your happiness is my happiness.
—Milton H. Erickson, M.D.

"**A**nd now we're going to play a game, and the main rule is that you can't move your feet. But you can move anything else, in any way you like. So let's start in 'Tadasana,' the Sacred Mountain Pose. And now wiggle your hips back and forth . . . And move in any way you like, just let your body be free, and follow any impulse to move, but keep your feet planted! (All move, free style for awhile)

And I'm going to say some words, and continue to move in any way you like, as I say these words . . . (One breath)
Your happiness, is my happiness . . . (One breath)

If you do well, I have done well . . . (One breath)

Let us root for each other to branch out and learn new things . . . (One breath)

If you have been holding on to something for too long, you can let it go, and something new may grow . . . (One breath)

And slowly come to a stop, and come back to Tadasana the Mountain Pose, and shut your eyes, bow your head, and notice your wonderful breathing . . . (One breath)

And the Earth beneath you . . . (One breath)

As breath refreshes you anew,

Love flows between the earth and you . . . (Two breaths)

G. The Flow

1. A Sense of Flow

In this game, flowing movements are explored. The idea is just to get kids "in the flow" of connected movements with their own and each other's bodies.

Teacher: "Let's move around the room and first let's move like molasses. V-e-r-y slowly, and thick, a slow motion kind of flow . . . (All move around like molasses)
and notice each other, and move with each other, and let's move like sail boats floating on a lake . . . a nice, flowing breeze . . . you can feel it gently pushing you . . . an easy-going kind of flow . . . (One breath)
and the wind gets faster—feel the wind at your back—you can move faster, a graceful kind of flow . . . (One breath) and slower again . . . (One breath)
and come to a rest, and stay in once place, but let your upper part move . . . back and forth, a swaying kind of flow . . . (One breath)
and notice your breathing . . . notice the flow . . . (One breath)
and now move to your breathing, just follow your breath around the room, whatever that means to you . . . just flow . . . (Three breaths)
and you can move like a clear, cool, mountain stream . . . a quiet, rushing kind of flow . . . (Two breaths) and now be blown around by the wind that keeps changing directions and speed . . . and pay attention to where everybody is, and where everyone is going, and just go with the flow of each other . . . (Three breaths)
and you can stop and find a nice spot with a little space around it . . . and come back to *Tadasana*, Sacred Mountain Pose."

2. Flow and Glide

"And while you're standing still, your imagination can flow and glide. So let's think of things that flow, like a river, or glide, like a bird, or maybe slide, like someone slipping on a banana peel. Can you think of anything that flows, or glides? Or slides?
(Teacher notes down, or remembers suggestions from class.)
And you can shut your eyes, and imagine the beautiful flow of a river . . . (Two breaths)
And you can imagine a flowing dancer . . . (Two breaths)
And can you imagine a gliding . . .

And now you can open your eyes and let your eyes flow around the room . . .
(Everyone looks around)

And now, staying together, let's flow like a river. Move in any way you like, but stay together." (All move together imagining a river. Following this, the teacher can create movement using other ideas that have been suggested and imagined, with the urging to stay together.)

And now, come to a stop, and return to Sacred Mountain Pose, and you can bow your head, and shut your eyes, and your heart is beating, your blood is flowing, and you can just notice the flow of thoughts and images and pictures. And you can notice the flow of time. And is time moving fast or slowly right now?" (A few breaths)

H. Final Relaxation (*Savasana)*

Teacher: "So let's get back to Earth, and return to Relaxation Pose. And you can lie down softly on your back, feet out hip distance apart, and you can let them flop out, your arms a few inches from your sides, palms pointed up . . . (One breath)

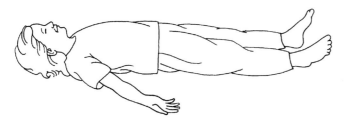

Savasana

"And make sure your spine is in line with your chin, and the top of your head. And the original word for this Relaxation Pose is,"*Savasana*," and notice the softness of the word, (*sha VA sah nah*). And let's work from the top to bottom, relaxing from your brain, down to your toes. And please don't work at this, because relaxation is the opposite of work. Just let your mind float, and your body will follow, floating on a quiet cloud . . . (One breath)

And imagine a candle, warming with a gentle glow, and let your jaw relax, like melting wax . . . (One breath)

And let that relaxation spread all over your head . . . imagine a pillow, comfortable, safe, gentle . . . relax your head, put it to bed . . . (One breath)

And they say "Well begun is half done." And paying attention to what you're doing is a good way to begin..and pay attention to your breathing . . . and let it be soft, and quiet . . .
(One breath)

And we could also say, 'Well done is well begun.' And imagine someone who has studied hard and really paid attention, and now it's time to let the mind play . . . and let tension and responsibility slide off your shoulders . . . like a stream, washing over boulders . . . (One breath) And your bones are a living, growing part of you, and old bone will be replaced by new growing bone. And relax your spine, and all your bones, all connected like telephones. (One breath)

And imagine two friends who had a fight . . . but their friendship is much bigger than that, and they have forgiven all in their hearts . . . (One breath)

Relax your chest, let it rest . . . (One breath)

And sometimes we hold ourselves very tight, and that's fine sometimes, but don't forget to remember to let go . . . (One breath)

Relax your hips, release their grips . . . (One breath)

And let relaxation travel down your legs and knees, calves, ankles, and let us understand that our feet bear the weight of your whole body when you stand, walk, run, and carry . . . so that NOW they can enjoy this wonderful rest . . . (One breath)

And you might want to thank your feet . . . (One breath)

And the floor they meet . . . (One breath)

And deeper still, let's thank the earth . . . (One breath) and deeper yet, let's thank your birth . . . (A few breaths)

And when you're ready, more fully rested, alert, awake, alive, you can open your eyes, and sit up, and notice how you feel."

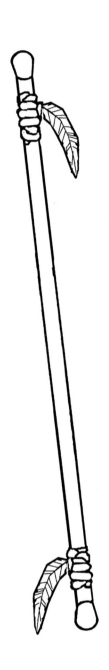

144

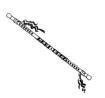

IV. SOLA Stikk Yoga

A. Introduction

1. History of SOLA Stikk Yoga

Sticks are useful to us in many ways—in athletics, in recreation, and in tools to name a few. We use sticks in hockey, fishing, baseball, pole vaulting, golf, lacrosse, and rowing. Think of just a few more places we find sticks: lollipops, shovels, flag poles, pogo sticks, writing implements, archery, and even chop sticks.

Yoga is one of the oldest forms of movement, and the incorporation of a stick into a yoga practice gives it a modern day twist. Nicole thought of using a stick as a yoga prop as she was cross-country skiing one winter's day in the Rocky Mountains and began to use her ski pole to do some yoga stretches. The SOLA Stikk was developed to help people hold poses longer, find intuitive alignment, and deepen their stretches. The SOLA Stikk can also serve as an individual totem, or an artistic expression of qualities or values one wants to incorporate into everyday life.

SOLA Stikk

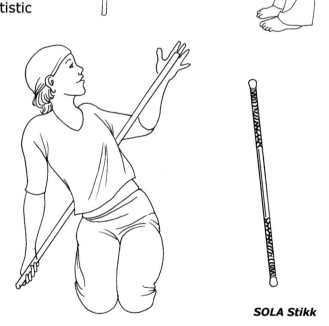

SOLA is an acronym for (S) Self-awareness, (O) Observation, (L) Love and (A) Acceptance. Nicole developed SOLA Stikk yoga as a way to build self-esteem, confidence, focus, awareness, and physical health in her students of all ages and abilities.

SOLA Stikk

2. The SOLA Stikk

   The actual stick can be as simple as a broom stick or a 3/4 inch dowel from a hardware store with a rubber stopper on the end or as imaginative as individual flare invites. The symbolism of a self-designed stick can be woven into the exercise to stand for courage, strength, focus, discipline, or fun. The process of creating of an individualized SOLA Stikk offers an outlet for individual creativity as well as a physical reminder of what a yoga practice can represent in a person's life.

3. Creating a SOLA Stikk*

   a. Women cancer survivors at retreats for Women Beyond Cancer decorated their SOLA Stikks with such materials as small beads, pink feathers, pink paper, silver tassels, and gold cord. Stikks can also be wrapped in yarn or ribbon. Their sticks represented their victory over cancer and the strength they gained from surviving cancer.

   b. Mothers and daughters (or any parent/child or duo combination) each can decorate one half of each other's stick. The sharing of the activity sets the framework for the sharing and bonding that comes from doing a yoga practice together, especially the partner poses. Each person then has an artistic expression to take with her and to use at another yoga practice.

   c. For an eight week program, divide the stick into eight sections and decorate a new section each week. Such an activity adds to the sense of growth and accomplishment offered from a yoga practice.

   *We'd love to hear your ideas for making SOLA Stikks.
   Visit our website and email us your ideas.
   You could win a free book or a yoga mat!

4. Holding a SOLA Stikk

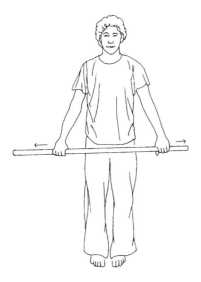

Pulling SOLA Stikk

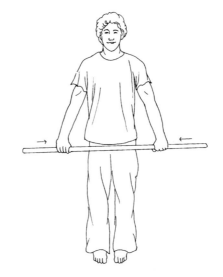

Pressing SOLA Stikk

By grasping the stick firmly between your strong hands, you can create a heating and energizing sensation in the middle of your body by pressing your hands together firmly and then pulling apart. While you do this, feel the connection of your shoulders and feel the heat in your upper body. When you pull your hands apart, feel how your shoulder blades hug into your spine and your heart opens outward.

B. The SOLA Stikk Practice

1. SOLA Salutation A

a. Letter Y Pose: Mountain Pose *(Tadasana)* Variation

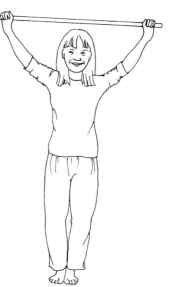

"In yoga, we always want to think about the breath. Your breath is rising up from your diaphragm, the muscle that sits below your lungs and above your belly button. Stand in Mountain Pose, your feet can be together or hip width apart. Begin to breathe in as your straighten your arms and raise the stick above your head to make the Letter Y.

Letter Y

Your legs and torso are the tail of your Y and your arms are the top. Can you make your letter Y taller by pressing your feet firmly into the ground and lifting your stick toward the sky? Lift and stretch from the waist, not just by stretching the arms. Feel how light and tall you can be when you roll the stick out to your fingertips. See yourself as a tree stretching higher to feel the sunshine and fresh air.

Begin to breathe out and then lower your stick as you bend your elbows. Let's do this two more times, as we begin with the inhale first, raising the stick and then lowering the stick when you exhale.

Benefits: This pose will encourage maximum lengthening through the body and will increase the blood flow to the heart and create more space for breath in the body.

b. Lowering Letter Y Touch Down: Mountain Pose *(Tadasana)* Variation

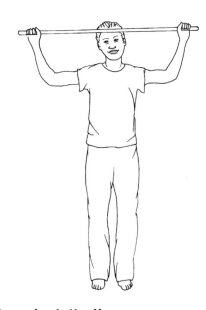

Lowering Letter Y

"As you start to breathe out, make believe the stick is squeezing all the air out of your lungs as it lowers all the way down so your arms are straight. Breathe in as you slowly lift the stick up, and then breathe out again as you lower it. Notice how you can match your movement with the breath moving in or out. Now this time imagine your chest slowly filling with air when the stick rises over your lungs. The stick is growing towards the sky and then your breath empties out when you lower the stick back down. Feel the strength between your hands as you press the ends of the stick together."

Benefits: The pushing/pulling sensation on the stick helps to build awareness of the muscular and skeletal structure in the upper body. Matching the breath with the movement of the stick will help integrate deeper breath awareness with physical movement—a key to a strong yoga practice and a powerful stress management technique.

c. Squatting Letter Y Pose: Chair Pose (Utkatasana) Variation

"After several rounds of combining the breathing/ pressing/pulling in Letter Y, bend your knees as if you are going to take a comfortable seat. Now breathe in and stretch up tall with your stick, keeping your heels on the ground. Hold this pose for a few breaths and feel the heat spreading through your leg muscles!"

Benefits: This pose helps to warm up the leg muscles (especially the quadriceps), allowing for a deeper stretch and strengthening the leg muscles. It also allows people to feel the isolation of movement between the upper body and lower body.

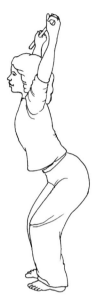

Squatting Letter Y

d. Saddle Pose: Chair Pose (Utkatasana) Variation

"From the letter Y press the stick across your thighs to find Saddle Pose. Straighten your arms so your palms press into the stick. Feel how your spine lengthens and makes a nice saddle so a little child could hop on your back and feel really secure. Your spine is rounded in and your belly button might be touching your thighs."

Benefits: Saddle pose lengthens the spine in a supported way and gives the lower body a rest. This pose also introduces the concept of using body parts with the stick to lengthen other body parts. All the muscles in the back are lengthened and toned in this pose. These include the latissimus dorsi, oblique, and trapezius muscles.

e. Tall Suspension Bridge: Half Down Dog Pose (Ardha Adho Mukha Svanasana)

"Take several deeper breaths and then extend the stick in front of you as though you are holding on to a trapeze bar and about to jump off the platform. You are reaching out with your strong spine, arms, and legs. After several more breaths, spin your

Saddle Pose

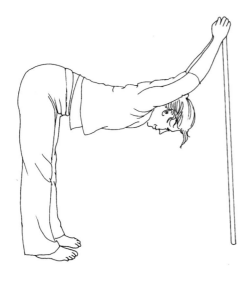

stick around and plant one end of it on the ground so it makes the top of a tall triangle— with your feet being the bottom two points of that triangle. Keep your hands towards the top of your stick and lengthen your head, neck and chest towards the ground—stretching long and strong like a suspension bridge. As you slowly straighten your legs and lift your hips toward the sky, feel the back of your legs (the hamstrings) start to release."

Benefits: Tall Suspension Bridge stretches the back of the legs without the intensity of a forward fold. It also helps find freedom and length through the thoracic cavity and opens up the heart. Gradual lengthening also occurs

Tall Suspension Bridge

between all of the vertebrae and the supporting muscles. The lower body also greatly benefits from this pose. The hamstrings gradually release and the ankles, calves and feet are strengthened and toned as well.

f. Tic Toc Letter Y: Crescent Moon Variation

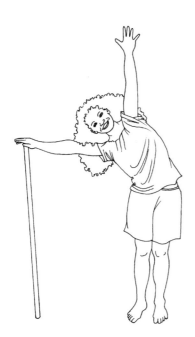

"Now our Letter Y is going to tic toc to each side of your body. Inhale your Y very tall and straight, as you exhale keep that length in your spine and lean over to the right. Inhale back to the top and then exhale over to the left. Now inhale again back to the top and this time release your stick by letting it slide through your hands with your body leaning over to the right. Plant your stick down arms length distance away with the bottom of your stick lined up with the middle of your right foot. You can push the stick away from you while keeping your arm straight.

Feel the stretch across the left side of your torso from your armpit down to your hip bone. Imagine your organs on the right side of your torso (liver, kidney, intestines) squish together. Extend your left arm to the sky and feel the blood and lymphatic fluid drain out of your arm. Keep your head in line with your spine and turn and look up to the sky. Take several breaths here, feeling your body stretch and come alive!

Tic Toc Letter Y

150

Now repeat on the left side, while you imagine the squeezing sponge, rinsing effect as the abdominal organs (pancreas, stomach, intestines, kidneys) are wrung out. After you stretch both sides, hang your body back into Tall Suspension Bridge and feel the length in your spine, between your ribs and through your side stomach muscles (obliques)."

Benefits: This pose lengthens the side of your body in a supported way. After stretching one side, it also serves as a way to feel the difference in the body before and after a pose. The pose lengthens the intercostal muscles (the tiny muscles between the ribs) and the muscles in the core. Tic Toc Letter Y also cleanses and tones the digestive organs. People are amazed at how differently their body feels after doing only one side. That sensation helps them realize how good SOLA Yoga Stikk makes their bodies feel.

2. SOLA Salutation B

a. Power Pendulum Pose: Lunge *(Anjenasana)* **Variation**

"Find your Letter Y and slowly bend your knees into Squatting Letter Y. Peel your left heel away from the floor, lifting the foot completely as you step back into a lunge. Rest your back knee, shin and top of the foot on the mat. Plant your stick down so it is across from your front big toe and lines up with your back knee. Holding on to the top of the stick, push it away from your body as you keep pressing your back knee on to the floor.

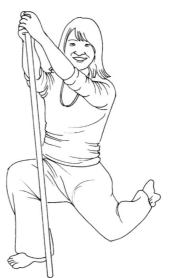

Exhale as you stretch forward and push the stikk away, and inhale as you release out of the stretch a little. Explore the rhythm of the breath and the movement as you exhale and stretch forward, inhale and release several times. Finish your power pendulum by extending out as far as you can."

Benefits: Nicole's high school rowing team loves to do this stretch before they get in their boats. The stikk supports them so they can explore more depth in this pose. Power Pendulum is a supported way to lengthen and strengthen the hip flexors (front of the hips) and quadricep muscles (top of the thigh).

Power Pendulum

b. Flag Pole Pose: Intense Side Stretch *(Parsvokonasana)* **Variation**

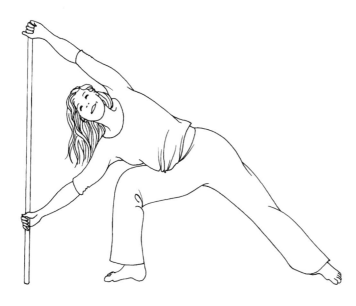

Flag Pole

"To find Flag Pole Pose, now rise up on to the ball of your back foot, lifting the back knee and straightening the back leg. Slowly begin to spin your back foot flat. Slide your right hand towards the bottom of the stick while your left hand is towards the top of the stick. Your chest, face and hips will be turning towards the side. It should feel like you are a flag hanging off of a flag pole. After holding this strengthening pose for several breaths, keeping your upper body still and finding your core strength, lift your torso up into the Y position with your hips and shoulders facing the side. Your body will be in a Warrior II position with the stick overhead. Your body position should look like the Letter X with the front knee bent and the front toes facing forward"

Note: This pose can be done with a partner by standing across from each other and sharing the stikk. The partners can pull against each other helping to lengthen and support each other. Nicole walks around gently pulling the top of a person's stick to challenge their balance.

Benefits: Flag Pole Pose lengthens one side of the body as it strengthens the other side. It also challenges the mind to find focus and balance in both the mind and the body. Using the stick as a leverage tool helps to lengthen the stretching side body more deeply.

c. Reverse Warrior 2 *(Virabhadrasana)* **Pose**

"Now wave your stick through the sky taking it side to side. Move with your breath as you exhale and reach forward over your knee, keeping your heart facing sideways. Inhale back up and then exhale towards your back straightened leg. Let's move with the breath three more times. Now extend your body over your back leg and release the stick so that it lines up with the middle of the back foot into Reverse Warrior.

Your back hand and extended arm will rest on the stick as a support. Your front knee is bent and your back leg is straight. Trace a rainbow across the sky with your front fingertips so your front arm and hand are reaching for the pot of gold towards that back arm. Hold this position for several breaths. Bring your body back up to Warrior II with a Letter Y upper body. Notice the difference you feel on one side of your body."

Benefits: Reverse Warrior with the stick strengthens the lower body while lengthening the upper body and strengthens and tones the kidneys and adrenal glands.

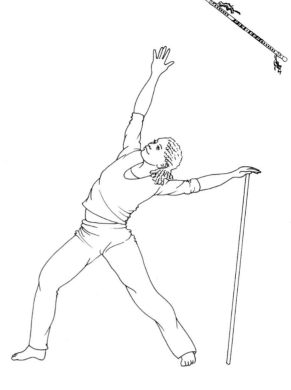

Reverse Warrior

d. Folded Letter X: Forward Fold Variation

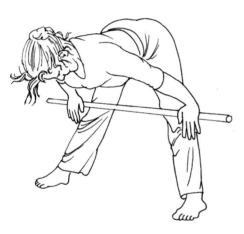

Folded Letter X

"We will repeat this on the other side, but first we need to make the Letter X with our bodies. From Warrior II, straighten the front leg and turn your front foot so it is parallel with your back foot. You are making the Letter X with your body. Reaching up high with your hands, sweep the stick halfway down as if you were going to fold your X in half . Lower the stick down so it presses against your lower thigh, above your knees. Press your arms straight with your hands on the outside of your knees.

Benefits: Folded Letter X helps us increase space between our vertebrae by using the stick and arms as a brace against the legs. When the stick is extended overhead while the body stays folded in half, deep core muscles are activated to hold this position.

e. Folded Letter X: Upside Down Pull

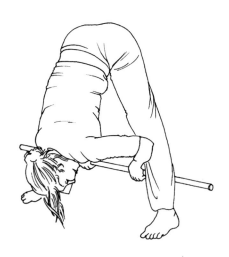

"Now release your body all the way into a forward fold. Weave the stick behind your lower legs and press the stick against the back of your legs. Try to pull your chin towards the stick as though you are doing a chin up. Feel the intense sensation in the back of your legs."

Benefits: This pose is an inversion, which increases blood flow to the brain. The upper body is strengthened by pulling the body towards the stick while the lower body is intensely lengthened. It's a perfect partnership!

Folded X: Upside Down Pull

f. Wide Suspension Bridge Pose: Wide Legged Half Down Dog
(Prasarita Ardha Adho Mukha Svanasana)

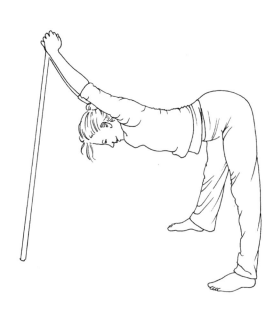

"This pose is similar to Tall Suspension Bridge Pose, but your feet are wide apart in a straddle. Hold your hands at the top of the stick and let your head and chest melt toward the ground. Relax into the pose for several breaths. To come out, press your stick against the top of your knees again to lengthen your spine as you raise your arms back to form the Letter Y. Continue rising up until you have moved into the Letter X."

Wide Suspension Bridge

3. Balancing Series

Now it is time to use the SOLA Stikk for its most obvious purpose—balance!

a. Tree Pose (*Vrksasana*)

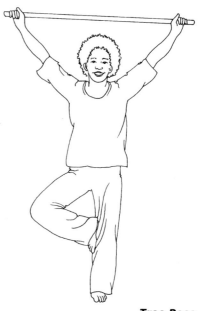

"Hold the stick in your left hand as a support and press the sole of your right foot against the inside of your left leg. We are making a tree. Slowly raise your stick overhead into the Letter Y. Grip your stick firmly with your hands to help you balance. Squeezing your hands towards each other will help you find the midline in your body which will help you balance. Hold here for several breaths, and then do the other side."

Benefits: Balance poses are always great ways to clear, calm, and challenge the mind. Using a stick gives people confidence while they play with the more challenging versions of Tree Pose. Squeezing the stick helps find the midline in the body.

Tree Pose

b. Drawbridge Pose

Note: Students love to stand across from each other and press the bottoms of their feet against each other for more support and partner focus. Maintaining eye contact is important when doing this pose.

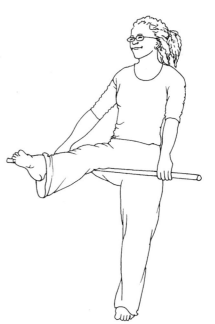

"To make a drawbridge from Tree Pose, hinge your right knee forward and weave your stick underneath the right thigh. Straighten your arms and let the stick support your lifted leg. Once you feel stable, lift your heart and straighten out the front leg so it looks like a drawbridge. For more of a challenge, try to keep your leg extended and release your stick overhead into the Letter Y."

Benefits: This pose helps a person sense the proportions in the body by using the full length of the arms and legs with the stick as a support. It also stretches the hamstrings and strengthens the legs.

Drawbridge

c. King Dancer Pose: (Natarajasana)

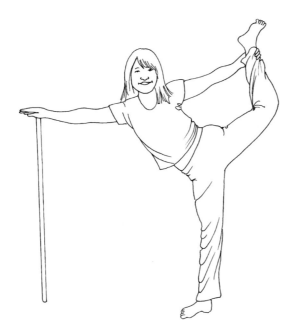

King Dancer

"From the Letter Y Pose, as you breathe in, raise your left foot and plant the stick in front of you for support. Reach behind you with your left hand and grasp the top of the foot. As you breathe out raise the back leg and kick your foot into your hand. Hold and enjoy this pose for several breaths. Come back to standing and take three rounds of breath. Repeat on the other side."

Challenge: Slowly lift the stick toward the sky so you are balancing only on your standing leg. Some students like the challenge of seeing how long and how high they can hold their leg. It challenges them to connect deeper to their bodies and gain more confidence.

Benefits: This pose opens up the hips and the chest, while it strengthens the standing leg. Using the stick to begin the pose, and then allowing the stick to release while still holding the pose, builds confidence and focus.

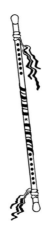

d. Number 4 Pose

Note: This pose is the ultimate multi-tasking pose. Students are challenged to balance, deeply stretch a very large muscle group while moving their bodies with their stick in a very foreign way. Athletes love the mental challenge of this pose and the deep stretch it provides.

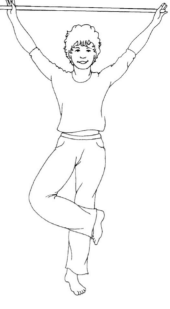

Number 4 Pose

"From Mountain Pose, shift your weight into the right foot and lift the left knee. Bring the left ankle to rest across the top of the right knee to make a Number 4 with your legs. Keep the left foot flexed, as if it were standing on the ground. Use your stick for balance. Once you feel steady, start to fold your upper body toward your knees.

Challenge yourself by lowering the stick and pressing it against the outside of the shin so it runs along the outside of your ankle, shin and knee. Then start to pull yourself upright bringing your bent leg with you. Slowly come out of the pose and back to Mountain Pose. Find your #4 on the other side."

Challenge: Flow from Number 4 to Tree Pose and back to Mountain Pose.

Benefits: This pose helps stretch the hip flexor muscles as well as strengthening the standing leg. It stretches the deep iliopsoas muscles, which run from the thoracic vertebra number 12 to the top of the femur. The mind is also challenged with this pose as we practice balancing and shifting of the weight.

4. Partner Poses

Partner poses are a wonderful way to build trust, to foster a sense of teamwork, and to develop communication skills. Working with a partner also develops awareness and focus as one has to pay attention to what the partner is doing. More importantly, partner poses make people smile, laugh, and have fun, thus reducing stress hormone levels and boosting the immune system.

a. Trusting Squats: Chair Pose Variation *(Utkatasana)*

"Find a partner that is about your size. Remember that in this pose you need to talk to each other so you can make adjustments and coordinate your movements. Stand across from each other so that you can both firmly hold the stick. Your feet need to be hip width apart (the outside of each foot lines up with the outside of the corresponding hip). You and your partner have to trust each other as you both breathe out and sit back on to your imaginary toadstool. Now lower down into a squatting position, maintaining that trust. It is important to keep all arms straight as though you were hanging from a trapeze bar. Practice taking a breath in together as you rise up, then exhaling together as you sit back. Do three more sets of coordinated breathing and trusting squats."

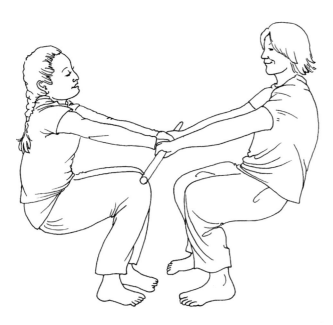

Caption: Trusting Squats

Benefits: Trusting Squats build communication skills and trust. In addition, it strengthens the quadriceps, lengthens the spine, and stretches the upper back and shoulders. It also increases flexibility in the ankles.

b. King Dancers *(Natarajasana)*

"Standing across from each other, each person holds the stick with his right hand and reaches back to grasp his left ankle with the left hand. Look directly into your partner's eyes to focus and find a shared strength. Now slowly raise the stick off the ground."

Challenge: Release the stick and grasp each other's right hands. To further the challenge, see how long each pair of King Dancers can hold their pose. The challenge will bring a calm to the room and a feeling of accomplishment and teamwork.

King Dancers

Benefits: This partner element of this pose is a fun and helpful way to get people to work together and to support each other as they focus on a single task. By adding the element of paired competition, people are tapping into deeper levels of mental clarity and teamwork.

c. Superman and Peter Pan

CAUTION!!

This pose must be done very slowly and with good communication between partners. The partners must be committed to listening to each other while the grounded partner is "flying". There is real danger that the standing partner pulls too hard on the stick and causes back injury to the person on the floor. Make certain to fully express these cautions to people before they do the pose. Anyone with lower back problems should NOT do this pose.

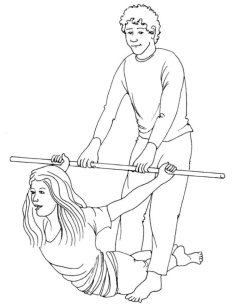

Superman and Peter Pan

"One person lie on your stomach, legs together, holding the stick in the extended arms behind you. Your partner stands with his feet on either side of your knees. He bends over and grasps the stick.

159

Breathe together as your partner says, "Inhale" and he slowly pulls and lifts the SOLA Stikk until you say, "Stop." Hold the stretch for two full breaths and slowly lower back to the mat. A slow release allows you the opportunity to strengthen the back muscles. Repeat one more time. Finish this pose by releasing the Stikk and moving, as if moving in slow motion, back into extended Child's Pose, with knees far apart and toes touching. Stay here for four breaths and switch places."

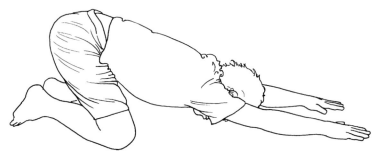

Note: Nicole teaches to yoga students who have all survived cancer, many of them breast cancer. This pose is an all-time favorite for them. Several of her students have felt intense positive emotional releases during this pose.

Extended Child's Pose

Benefits: This pose requires constant communication and trust between partners. The pose is excellent for stretching the entire front of the upper body and strengthening the lower back. The person "flying" lengthens the muscle groups on the front of the upper body. This pose strengthens and tones the muscles in the upper back. The standing partner also strengthens her legs, back, and arms.

5. Floor Work

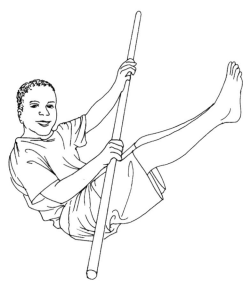

"Now that we have strengthened our lower backs, let's do some fun SOLA Stikk abdominal strengthening and stretching."

a. Paddling: Boat Pose (*Navasana*)

Nicole, a former collegiate competitive rower, developed this pose because water sports like rowing, kayaking and canoeing are so much fun.

"Start by holding the stick underneath your thighs. Let your arms straighten while your upper body releases back. Using your core, or stomach muscles, extend your legs out straight. Keep your legs straight as you bring the stick in front of your body so it feels like a paddle. Now

Paddling

use the stick as a paddle by taking it side to side making sweeping, paddling motions. Paddle 10 times on each side. Repeat this until your stomach muscles feel strong and alive."

Benefits: This pose is excellent for building core strength and balance. The paddling motion with the arms and hands also gently lubricates the shoulder joints, often a point of injury in people.

b. Pete's Pretzel: Simple Twist (Bharadvajasana I)

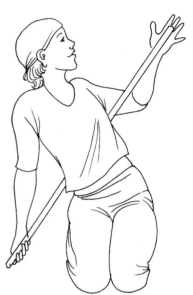

Pete's Pretzel

"Sit in a comfortable position and press the stick against your middle back, hooking it to the inside of your elbows and forearms. The end of the stick needs to be pressing against your palms. Tilt your stick over to one side and press the rubber stopper into the ground for stability. Walk your hand down to the rubber stopper. Your other hand will be pressing the palm against the top end of the stick. By pressing your palm against the stick, you will have leverage to turn your upper shoulder towards the stick. This should feel like the top side of your torso is turning open. Take several deep breaths holding this pose and then change sides by dropping the stick to the other side and readjusting your hands and shifting your weight."

Benefits: This pose is a good upper back release if you have a tendency to hunch over when you sit in a chair. It is excellent for opening up the chest and releasing the stress that is stored between the shoulder blades. The upper spine (thoracic and cervical vertebrae) benefit greatly because of the twisting effect of this pose.

c. Happy Baby Pose (Ananda Balasana)

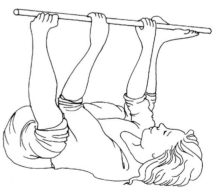

Happy Baby

"Lie on your back and gently draw your knees into your chest, keeping your knees apart. Press the stick against the bottom of your feet with your hands holding on to the stick between your knees. Roll the stick along the bottom of your feet, massaging them while you enjoy feeling like a happy baby."

Benefits: Happy Baby Pose opens the hips and stretches the bottoms of the feet, helping to keep the plantar fascia healthy.

6. The SOLA Circle

The image or symbol of a circle or wheel is found in many philosophies. One example is chakras, Sanskrit for "wheel" or "circle". Chakras are loosely defined as spinning wheels of energy serving to collect and distribute various life energies. Another image of the circle is the mandala, loosely translated from Sanskrit as "circle" or "center." The mandala pattern symbolizes the grand organizational design of life itself and our relationship to the infinite or the cosmos. The mandala is an archetypal symbol, also found in Native American art and rituals and in Christian cathedrals. Carl Jung brought the term mandala to modern usage employing the concept in healing art therapy.

So the idea of using a circle to practice yoga is simply a celebration and extension of these concepts of connections, community, flow, exploration of self, and circles. The SOLA Circle allows people to gain individual strength by working in a group. The various poses stretch and strengthen muscles, develop breathing awareness, and foster communication and group skills.

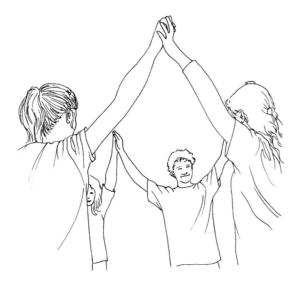

The SOLA Circle

a. The SOLA Circle

"We are going to use the power of the group to strengthen and lengthen our individual bodies. Let's make a circle so that you can press your palms against the palms of the people on either side. Your feet are spread so that the outside edges of your feet touch your neighbor's. Think about the largest living organism on the planet—a grove of aspens connected by their underground roots, all sharing energy and strength."

b. The Pointed Crown Press

"Keep your arms in the air with your fingertips reaching for the sky and let your head and chest gently move forward, stretching out your chest muscles. See how all our arms make points as our chests melt forward. Notice how pressing your palms against your neighbor's not only give you support and makes the whole circle strong."

162

Benefits: Pointed Crown Press stretches the pectoral muscles and opens the shoulders. Similar to Parachute Press, it requires trust and teamwork for proper execution.

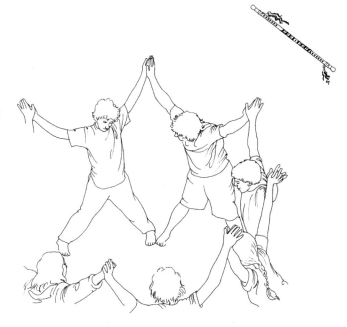

Pointed Crown Press

c. The SOLA Tree and SOLA Leg Fence

"Everyone find their Tree Pose standing on your right leg. Remember all trees can look and stand differently. You may have the sole of your left foot pressing into your right calf or right thigh (but not your knee). You can stabilize and support each other by holding each others arms as you balance as a group. Once you feel that everyone is stable, open up your hearts while keeping that foot on the inside of your leg."

Challenge: "Extend one leg to the side and grasp your neighbor's leg with the opposite hand. Feel how everyone is connected by holding on and lifting their neighbors' legs. The legs and arms have made a fence! This is called SOLA Leg Fence. Hold this side for three breaths and then switch sides."

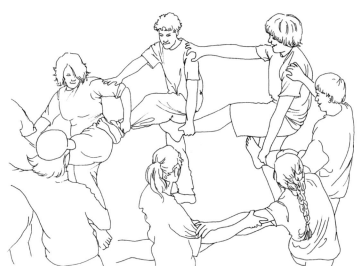

SOLA Circle Leg Fence

Benefits: The balancing poses develop group confidence and trust while strengthening the standing leg and lengthening the pectoral muscles) and hamstrings (SOLA Leg Fence). The group can be challenged further by trying to hold still without wobbling for as long as possible.

d. Number Four Pose

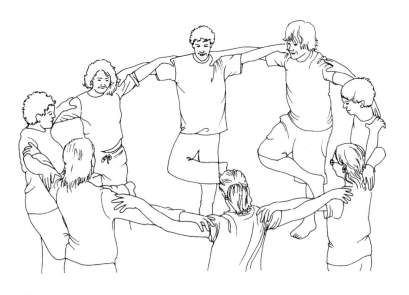

*SOLA Circle
Number Four*

"This pose is an especially challenging pose of trust and support. Release your legs back to standing. Cross the left ankle over the outside of the right knee so you make the Number 4. To keep your alignment, lift the left hip up and back. Now take a seat and feel your hips open. Feeling the strength and support from the group, slowly bend over toward your knees. Hold this for two breaths and then as you all inhale, lift your chest. We will do this sequence three times and return to standing, but keep holding on to your neighbors for balance."

Note: This pose builds team spirit. Nicole's rowing team loves the challenge of this pose because they all have to work together as though working together in a boat.

e. Rockette's Kick

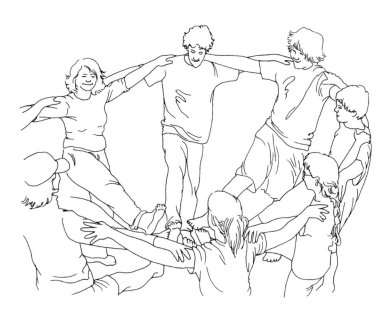

SOLA Circle Rockette Kick

"With your arms still around your neighbors, as a group, kick your leg out as high as you can and hold the pose. Point all toes to the middle of the circle. As a group, change the direction of your leg so it swings behind the group. With arms still interlaced, tilt your upper bodies forward, while extending your legs behind you in a ballet dancer's arabesque."

Note: To make a coordinated flow, while developing leadership skills and teamwork skills, have a designated leader call out a direction for all to kick their legs: to the front, to the left, to the right, or to the back. Expect a lot of giggling and laughter during this pose.

Benefits: This pose is excellent for building length and strength in both of the legs. It also builds teamwork, leadership, balance, and mental clarity.

f. SOLA Stikk Weave

"Now we are ready for a more trusting activity incorporating SOLA Stikk into the circle. Create the SOLA Circle again with the outside edges of your feet touching while holding your SOLA stick. Transition carefully with your neighbors, exchanging ends of each stick so you actually end up holding one end of each stick and not your own. The challenge is, as a team, is to recreate all the previous SOLA Circle poses without dropping any of the sticks."

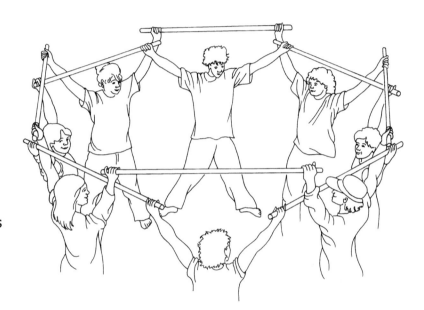

SOLA Stikk Weave

Final Note: Perhaps by introducing kids and teens to yoga . . . they can remember years later . . . a certain something . . . that made them feel a certain way, not really sure what or why, but just enough to give them the idea to try yoga . . . and perhaps find some centering in their lives.

As St. Augustine said,
Since you cannot do good to all, you are to pay special attention to those who, by accidents of time, or place, or circumstance, are brought into closer connection with you.

NAMASTE

REFERENCES

1) Folan, Lilias. *Lilias! Yoga Gets Better With Age*. Rodale Press. 2006. p. 7.

2) Desikachar, T.K.V. *The Heart of Yoga: Developing a Personal Practice*. Inner Traditions. 1999. p. 5.

3) Bell, Charlotte. *Mindful Yoga, Mindful Life: A Guide for Everyday Practice*. Berkeley: Rodmell Press. 2007. p. 16.

4) Iyengar, B.K.S. *Yoga: The Path to Holistic Health*. New York: Dorling Kindersley Limited. 2001. p. 21.

5) Hatfield, Elaine, and Cacioppo, John. *Emotional Contagion*. Cambridge: Cambridge University Press. 1993.

6) Lasater, Judith Hanson, Ph.D., P.T. *30 Essential Yoga Poses.* Berkeley: Rodmell Press. 2003. p. 7.

7) Fraley, Barbara and Arthur Aron, "The Effect of Shared Humorous Experience on Closeness in Initial Encounters," *Personal Relationships* 11 (2004) pp. 61-78.

8) Goleman, Daniel. *Social Intelligence*. New York: Bantam Books. 2006. pp. 44-45.

9) Rimer, Sara. "Less Homework, More Yoga, From Principal that Hates Stress." *The New York Times*. October 29, 2007.

10) Website for GreenTREE Yoga: www.greentreeyoga.org.

11) Jenkins, Lee. "A Twist on Preparation Wins Converts". *New York Times*. February 12, 2007.

12) Mohan, A. G. *Yoga for Body, Breath, and Mind.* Boston: Shambhala. 1993. p. 31.

13) Farhi, Donna. *The Breathing Book: Good Health and Vitality Through Essential Breath Work*. New York: Henry Holt Company. 2003. p. xvi

14) Payne, Larry, Ph.D. and Richard Usatine, M.D. *Yoga Rx: A Step-by-Step Program to Promote Health, Wellness, and Healing for Common Ailments*. New York: Random House. 2002. p. 38

15) McCall, Timothy, M.D. *Yoga as Medicine: The Yogic Prescription for Health and Healing*. New York: Bantam Books. 2007. p. 30

16) Gladwell, Malcolm. *The Tipping Point: How Little Things Can Make a Big Difference*. New York: Little, Brown and Company. 2002. p. 126-127.

17) Lasater. p. 11.

18) Goleman, Daniel. *Social Intelligence: The New Science of Human Relationships*, New York: Bantam Books. 2007. p. 44.

17) Payne. p. 29.

SANSKRIT PROUNCIATIONS

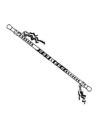

Asana: (AHS-anna**)** *asana*=**seat**

Bow pose: *Dhanurasana.* (don-your-AHS-anna) *dhanu*=bow

Bridge Pose: *Setu Bandha* (SET-too BAHN-dah) *setu*=dam, dike, or bridge
   bandha=lock

Butterfly: (Bound Angle Pose): *Baddha Konasana.*(BAH-dah cone-AHS-anna)
baddha=bound ; *kona*=angle

Chair Pose: *Utkatasana* (OOT-kah-TAHS-anna)
Utkata=powerful, fierce

Child's Pose: *Balasana.* (bah-LAHS-anna). *Bala*=child

Cobra Pose: *Bhujangasana.* (boo-jang-GAHS-anna). *Bhujanga*=serpent, snake

Crow (also known as Crane): Bakasana *(bahk-AHS-anna) baka*=crane

Downward-Facing Dog. *Adho Mukha Svanasana. (AH-doh MOO-kah shvah-*
   NAHS-   anna) adho=downward; *mukha*=face;*svana*=dog

Eagle Pose: *Garudasana* (gah-rue-DAHS-anna) Garuda=the mythic "king of the
   birds,"

Final Relaxation *Savasana: (shah-VAHS-anna) sava*=corpse

Fish Pose: *Matysasana* (mot-see-AHS-anna*) matsya*=fish

Flat Back: *Ardha Uttana*sana (are-dah oot-tan-AHS-anna)
   ardha = half ; uttana = intense stretch

Forward Bend (standing): *Uttanasana* (OOT-tan-AHS-ahna*)*
utt=intense; *tan*-to stretch or extend

Half Handstand: *Ardha Adho Mukha Vrksasana*
   (are-dah ah-doh moo-kah vriks-SHAHS-anna) Ardha=half; *adho mukha* = face
   downward (adho = downward; mukha = face) ; *vrksa* = tree

Half Moon Pose: *Ardha Chandrasana . (are-dah chan-DRAHS-anna)*
Ardha=half; *candra*=glittering, shining, having the brilliancy or hue of light (said of
   the gods); usually translated as "moon"

Half Shoulderstand: *Ardha Sarvangasana (ARE-dah sar-van-GAHS-anna)*

King Dancer or Lord of the Dance Pose. *Natarajasana (not-ah-raj-AHS-anna)*
Nata=actor, dancer, mime *raja*=king

Mountain Pose: *Tadasana.* (*tah-DAHS-anna*) *tada*=mountain.

Prayer Pose: *Anjali Mudra* (Salutation Seal). *Anjali*=a gesture of reverence, salutation *mudra*=seal (The gesture "seals" energy in the body)

Pretzel Pose or Half Lord of the Fishes Pose: *Ardha Matsyendrasana.* (ARE-dah MOT-see-en-DRAHS-anna*) ardha*=half. *Matsyendra*=king of the fish; *matsya*=fish; *indra*=ruler

Rainbow Pose: Vasisthasana (vah-sish-TAHS-anna*)* *Vasistha*=literally means "most excellent, best, richest."

Side Crow*: Parsva Bakasana. (parsh-voh- bahk-AHS-anna) parsva*=side, flank;*)* *baka* =crane

Tree Pose: *Vrksasana (*vrik-SHAHS-anna*) vrksa*=tree
Upward-Facing Dog:Urdhva Mukha Svanasana. (ERD-vah MOO-kah shvon-AHS-anna) urdhva mukha=face upward; urdhva=upward; mukha=face; svana=dog

Simple Twist: *Bharadvajasana I (bah-ROD-va-JAHS-anna),Bharadvaja*=one of seven legendary seers, credited with composing the hymns collected in the *Vedas*

Warrior 1, 2, and 3: Virabhadrasana 1, 2, and 3. (veer-ah-bah-DRAHS-anna) *Virabhadra* = the name of a fierce warrior, an incarnation of Shiva,

*Special Thanks to **Yoga Journal** for use of these pronounciations/definitions. More information available at: http://www.yogajournal.com/poses/finder/browse_index

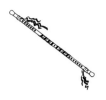

ABOUT THE AUTHORS AND THE ILLUSTRATOR

Yael Calhoun, M.A., M.S.

Yael is the Executive Director of GreenTREE Yoga, a nonprofit committed to presenting yoga as a life-long tool for physical and emotional health to young people and adults in a variety of settings, including schools, camps, senior centers, clubs, correctional facilities, and shelters. Yael has studied and practiced yoga for over 15 years. In addition to teaching adult yoga, she also teaches yoga to youth and young adults at shelters, summer camps, boys' and girls' clubs, to the disabled, and wherever she is invited.

Yael's education includes a B.A. from Brown University, as well as a Master's Degree in Education from Southern Connecticut State University and a Master's Degree in Natural Resources Science from the University of Rhode Island. Her job experiences include teaching in the classroom, both at the college level and the primary school level, working as a municipal environmental planner, and teaching yoga. Yael also is the author of almost a dozen books.

Yael is the co-author of *Create a Yoga Practice for Kids: Fun, Flexibility and Focus* by Yael Calhoun and Matthew R. Calhoun (Sunstone Press, 2006), a book Lilias Folan calls the "Best children's yoga book on the market today. Excellent descriptions, delightful illustrations." Judith Hanson Lasater says it is "an inspiring and upbeat book that will not only charm children but also educate and support their teachers."

Yael enjoys life at the base of the Rocky Mountains in Salt Lake City with her husband, Patrick A. Tresco, and their three sons, Sam (13), Ben (12), and Alex (11). They love to ski, mountain bike, hike, and kayak and are learning to rock climb.

Matthew R. Calhoun, C.E.Ht

Matthew R. Calhoun is a certified children's yoga teacher and holds three certifications in hypnotherapy. He created yoga programs for children at the Chicago Yoga Institute, and at Onward Neighborhood House, a settlement house for inner city children and teenagers. He is a practicing Certified Ericksonian Hypnotherapist, working with clients individually and in groups. He uses yogic techniques such as breathing, body awareness, movement and meditation to facilitate relaxation and an openness to healing communication, combining these techniques with alternative healing modalities such as hypnotherapy and Therapeutic Touch. He has taught physicians at the Weill Medical College of Cornell University Therapeutic Touch and mind/body communication for use with their patients.

The many groups he has served include disabled people, low-income single mothers, stressed-out social workers, people with substance abuse histories, people with HIV, homeless people and elderly people dealing with anxiety and depression. In 2004, he started a Healing-Group at the One-Stop Wellness Center in New York. In 2001, he was honored as an outreach practitioner by Healing Works in Manhattan for generosity of spirit. Matthew is the co-author of *Create a Yoga Practice for Kids* (Sunstone Press, 2006).

Nicole Hamory

Nicole's introduction to Yoga began after an intense relationship with her body as a Division I rower. Her body was riddled with pain, injury and discomfort. Yoga quickly became a physical healing tool as well as a spiritual necessity. Nicole began teaching yoga to current and former Olympians (members of the National Rowing Team) and the Northeastern University Crew in Boston before moving to Utah.

Nicole is the Program Director of GreenTREE Yoga, a nonprofit committed to presenting yoga as a life-long tool for physical and emotional health to young people and adults in a variety of settings, including schools, camps, senior centers, clubs, correctional facilities, and shelters. She created SOLA Stikk Yoga (patent pending), a style of yoga that incorporates a stick to enable a person to hold poses longer, balance and find proper alignment. The stick is also an artistic expression piece as people create their own "totems".

Nicole has studied and practiced yoga for the past 10 years. She is a certified D'ana Baptiste yoga instructor, with a strong influence and trainings from Baron Baptiste, Ana Forrest and Anusara Yoga (Adam Ballenger). Nicole currently teaches in a variety of settings in the Salt Lake City area: at colleges, schools, ski resorts, juvenile detention centers, the men's jail and women's prison, and the Huntsman Cancer Institute. She also teaches many classes for the disabled in a variety of settings and works with Women Beyond Cancer. In addition, Nicole brings yoga to her weekly high school rowing team as part of their cross training (Utah Junior Crew).

Nicole's education includes a B.A. from Rutgers College in Elementary Education and American Studies, as well as coursework toward an M.Ed. in Marriage and Family Therapy program at the University of Massachusetts/Boston. Her passions include developing and teaching motivational wellness programs for youth-at-risk and college students. In her spare time, Nicole loves to do anything in nature with friends, family and her beloved dog, Laszlo.

Carol Anne Coogan

Carol Coogan is an artist, illustrator, graphic designer and writer. Carol has over twenty years of commercial creative service experience and fine art exhibition. She writes and illustrates a weekly newspaper column called the *Backyard Naturalist*. Other books illustrated by Carol Coogan are *Create a Yoga Practice For Kids* by Yael Calhoun and Matthew Calhoun (Sunstone Press, 2006), *2008 Magical Almanac* and *2009 Magical Almanac* (Llewellyn Publications), and *Way of Water* by Lee Welles (Chelsea Green). Carol has also published a first year compilation of her newspaper column, *Backyard Naturalist*, which she wrote and illustrated.

RESOURCES

1. *Yoga as Medicine* by Timothy McCall, M.D. (Bantam Books. 2007)

2. *Mindful Yoga, Mindful Life* by Charlotte Bell (Rodmell Press. 2007)

3. *Lilias! Yoga Gets Better With Age* by Lilias Folan (Rodale Press, 2006)

4. *30 Essential Yoga Poses* by Judith Hanson Lasater (Rodmell Press, 2003)

5. *The Complete Idiot's Guide to Kids' Yoga* by Jodi Komitor. (Alpha, 2000)

6. *The Yoga of Breath.* By Richard Rosen. (Shambhala, 2002)

7. *Yoga Rx: A Step-by-Step Program to Promote Health, Wellness, and Healing for Common Ailments.* By Larry Payne, Ph.D. and Richard Usatine, M.D. (Random House. 2002).

31901050534132

Breinigsville, PA USA
20 March 2011
258011BV00001B/37/P

9 780865 346864